Case Studies to Accompany

Bates' Guide to Physical Examination and History Taking

NINTH EDITION

Case Studies to Accompany

Bates' Guide to Physical Examination and History Taking

NINTH EDITION

Fiona R. Prabhu, MD
Assistant Professor, Family and Community Medicine
Texas Tech University Health Sciences Center
Lubbock, Texas

Lynn S. Bickley, MD
Professor, Internal Medicine and Neuropsychiatry
Associate Dean for Curriculum, School of Medicine
Texas Tech University Health Sciences Center
Lubbock, Texas

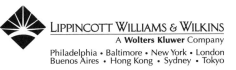

LIPPINCOTT WILLIAMS & WILKINS
A **Wolters Kluwer** Company
Philadelphia • Baltimore • New York • London
Buenos Aires • Hong Kong • Sydney • Tokyo

Acquisitions Editor: Elizabeth Nieginski
Ancillary Editor: Doris S. Wray
Production Editor: Audrey Lickwar
Director of Nursing Production: Helen Ewan
Senior Managing Editor/Production: Erika Kors
Creative Director: Doug Smock
Manufacturing Coordinator: Karin Duffield
Compositor: TechBooks
Printer: Victor Graphics

9th Edition

15 14 13 12 11

ISBN: 0-7817-9221-5

Care has been taken to confirm the accuracy of the information presented and to
describe generally accepted practices. However, the authors, editors, and publisher are
not responsible for errors or omissions or for any consequences from application of
the information in this book and make no warranty, express or implied, with respect
to the content of the publication.

The authors, editors, and publisher have exerted every effort to ensure that drug
selection and dosage set forth in this text are in accordance with the current
recommendations and practice at the time of publication. However, in view of
ongoing research, changes in government regulations, and the constant flow of
information relating to drug therapy and drug reactions, the reader is urged to
check the package insert for each drug for any change in indications and dosage
and for added warnings and precautions. This is particularly important when the
recommended agent is a new or infrequently employed drug.

Some drugs and medical devices presented in this publication have Food and Drug
Administration (FDA) clearance for limited use in restricted research settings. It is the
responsibility of the health care provider to ascertain the FDA status of each drug or
device planned for use in his or her clinical practice.

Preface

This case book, which accompanies *Bates' Guide to Physical Examination and History Taking, ninth edition*, is designed to help students apply their skills in history taking and physical examination to actual case vignettes and to test their knowledge and skills by answering case-based questions. By working through the cases, students can begin to integrate information from health histories and examinations and develop tools for clinical reasoning and assessment. These steps, in turn, will aid students in formulating hypotheses leading to reasonable sets of differential diagnoses. The case book is written with the assumption that students have had basic courses in human anatomy and physiology as well as some experience with patient care.

In general, the chapters in the case book are aligned with those in *Bates' Guide to Physical Examination and History Taking, ninth edition*. Most chapters in this case book begin with a case study featuring a chief complaint and brief history of present illness. Students are asked to identify the parts of the physical examination they would choose to perform, based on the history that is given. Next, students read the actual physical examination findings. After receiving all the information, students develop three possible diagnoses.

In addition to case studies, some chapters contain multiple choice, matching, or labeling exercises, and sometimes a combination of all three. These exercises are related to the chapter's topic and are based on information that can be found in *Bates' Guide to Physical Examination and History Taking, ninth edition*. Answers to all of the exercises can be found at the end of this case book.

Please note that Chapter 16 of this case book, "The Pregnant Woman," does not contain a case study because students would need a more advanced knowledge base and more clinical experience to work through a case on this subject to develop differential diagnoses. For this chapter, multiple choice and matching exercises are provided.

We hope that this case book will be a useful tool for students seeking to develop their clinical reasoning and differential diagnosis skills and that it achieves its primary goal of helping students to become more comfortable with integrating information when presented with real patients.

Fiona R. Prabhu, MD
Lynn S. Bickley, MD

Contents

Abbreviations

AP	anterior–posterior
BP	blood pressure
bpm	beats per minute
CN	cranial nerve
CVA	costovertebral angle
EOMs	extraocular movements
GxPx	gravida (number of pregnancies); parity (number of births)
HR	heart rate
JVP	jugular venous pressure
KOH	potassium hydroxide
MCL	midclavicular line
MCP	metacarpophalangeal
PIP	proximal interphalangeal
PMI	point of maximal intensity
RAMs	rapid alternating movements
RCM	right costal margin

CHAPTER 1

Beginning the Physical Examination: General Survey and Vital Signs

■ Case Study: Fever, Adult

CHIEF COMPLAINT: "I have a fever that won't go away."

History of Present Illness:
Cindy is a 27-year-old photographer who presents for evaluation of fever. The fever started 10 days ago. She states that the fever comes and goes—it lasts for 30–60 minutes; she takes Tylenol and it gets better, but then it comes back after 4 hours. She has measured her temperature; the highest was 101.5°F and the lowest was 100.4°F.

She denies any sick contacts. She has lost her appetite and has been trying to drink more fluids to avoid dehydration. She has lost 10 pounds. She has a throbbing headache that seems to linger after the fever goes down and some neck soreness. She denies changes in her vision or her hearing, but her ears hurt. She has a sore throat and increased drainage out of her nose as well as nasal congestion. She has pain in her face and in her teeth. She has a cough but denies any sputum production. She has no chest pain or palpitations. She has no abdominal pain, diarrhea, dysuria, pelvic pain, or vaginal discharge. She has no swelling in her legs. She has soreness in the muscles all over her body, and even her scalp hurts. She has pain in her wrists, shoulders, hips, knees, and ankles.

She had chicken pox at age 8 but was otherwise healthy. She has never been hospitalized. She has never been pregnant. She is sexually active and has had six lifetime partners. She takes birth control pills. She lives alone. She smokes cigarettes occasionally, drinks alcohol socially, and denies illicit drug use.

Her parents are healthy.

What parts of the exam would you like to perform? (Circle the appropriate areas.)

General Survey	Breasts and Axillae
Vital Signs	Female Genitalia
Skin	Male Genitalia
Head and Neck	Anus, Rectum, and Prostate
Thorax and Lungs	Peripheral Vascular/Extremities
Cardiovascular	Musculoskeletal
Abdomen	Nervous System

What physical findings are you looking for to help determine the diagnosis?

These are the actual findings on physical examination:

General Survey	Patient is an alert, young woman, sitting comfortably on the examination table
Vital Signs	BP 85/55 mm Hg; HR 110 bpm and regular; respiratory rate 14 breaths/min; temperature 100.9°F
Skin	No rash
HEENT	Normocephalic, atraumatic
	Sclera white, conjunctivae clear; pupils constrict from 4 mm to 2 mm and are equal, round, and reactive to light and accommodation; fundi with sharp discs
	External ear canals pink; tympanic membranes dull with retraction bilaterally
	Nose patent with edematous erythematous turbinates
	Face tender to palpation in the maxillary sinuses, worse on the left than on the right
	Oropharynx moist with erythema in the posterior pharyngeal wall; no exudates
	Neck supple with tender, enlarged (1-2 cm) anterior cervical lymph nodes; neck with full range of motion
Cardiovascular	Good S1, S2; no S3, S4; no murmurs or extra sounds
Lungs	Breath sounds vesicular; no wheezes, rales, or rhonchi
Abdomen	Bowel sounds active; soft, nontender to palpation; nondistended
Musculoskeletal	Full range of motion; no swelling or deformity; muscles with normal bulk and tone

Based on this information, what is your differential diagnosis?

1. _____

2. _____

3. _____

■ Case Study: Unexplained Weight Loss

CHIEF COMPLAINT: "I keep losing weight."

History of Present Illness:
Ms. L., a 25-year-old retail store manager, comes to your office because of continued weight loss over the past 2 months. She has lost 25 pounds and denies intentional weight loss. She states that she is eating the same amount of food as before the weight loss. She has noticed night sweats and subjective fevers; her hair is falling out; she does experience some episodes of palpitations; and she feels physically weaker since losing weight. She has had increased stress at home and at work. She has had decreased energy and concentration, with episodes of crying and sadness because of a sense of helplessness in dealing with these stressors. She reports no headaches, visual changes, chest pain or pressure, or abdominal pain. She denies wanting to hurt herself or others. She does not hear voices.

She does not smoke, drink, or use illicit drugs. She has worked at her present position for the last 3 years and is coming up for promotion soon. She has been married for 7 years and has two children. She denies living in a situation where she is emotionally, physically, or sexually abused.

Her medical history is unremarkable. She had an appendectomy at age 8 and a tonsillectomy at age 4.

Her mother and grandmother have had depression but are otherwise healthy; her father has hypertension.

What parts of the exam would you like to perform? (Circle the appropriate areas.)

General Survey	Breasts and Axillae
Vital Signs	Female Genitalia
Skin	Male Genitalia
Head and Neck	Anus, Rectum, and Prostate
Thorax and Lungs	Peripheral Vascular/Extremities
Cardiovascular	Musculoskeletal
Abdomen	Nervous System

What physical findings are you looking for to help determine the diagnosis?

These are the actual findings on physical examination:

General Survey	Alert, young woman with an expressionless face and monotonous tone of voice; resting comfortably on the examining table
Vital Signs	BP 114/67 mm Hg; HR 82 bpm and regular; respiratory rate 18 breaths/min; temperature 98.8°F
Skin	No rash
HEENT	Normocephalic, atraumatic
	Pupils equal, round, and reactive to light and accommodation; constrict from 5 mm to 2 mm
	Disc margins are sharp; fundi without hemorrhages or exudates
	External ear canals patent; tympanic membranes with good cone of light
	Oral mucosa pink, without enlarged tonsils; dentition good; pharynx without exudates
Neck	Supple, without thyromegaly; no lymphadenopathy
Thorax and Lungs	Thorax symmetric with good expansion
	Lungs resonant; breath sounds vesicular
Cardiovascular	JVP 6 cm above right atrium; carotid upstrokes brisk, without bruits
	PMI tapping and nondisplaced
	Good S1, S2; no S3, S4; no murmurs
Peripheral Vascular/ Extremities	Calves supple without edema; peripheral pulses are 2+ bilaterally
Musculoskeletal	Full range of motion in all joints, no swelling or deformities
Neurologic	Mental status: Patient is oriented to person, place, and time
	Cranial nerves: CN II through XII intact
	Motor: Good bulk and tone, strength 5/5 throughout
	Cerebellar: RAMs, finger to nose, and heel to shin intact; gait with normal base
	Sensory: Pinprick and light touch intact and symmetric throughout
	Reflexes: 2+ and symmetric throughout, with toes downgoing
	Folstein Mini-Mental Status score: 28/30

Based on this information, what is your differential diagnosis?

1. _____

2. _____

3. _____

■ Multiple Choice

Choose the single best answer.

1. All of the following parameters are vital signs EXCEPT:
   (A) Pulse
   (B) Respiratory rate
   (C) Blood pressure
   (D) Abdominal girth

2. A 55-year-old woman with a known history of moderately severe congestive heart failure presents to the emergency room for evaluation of progressive shortness of breath. She ran out of her medications 1 week ago. Upon general survey of this patient, who is in acute congestive heart failure, you would expect to see her:
   (A) Sitting up
   (B) Supine
   (C) Laying on her left side
   (D) Standing

3. A 66-year-old man with a known history of chronic obstructive pulmonary disease (COPD) presents to the clinic for evaluation of progressive shortness of breath. He had an upper respiratory infection 2 weeks ago, and the symptoms have gotten worse. On physical examination, you find that he is having an acute exacerbation of his COPD. On general survey of this patient, you would expect to see him:
   (A) Sitting up and leaning forward with arms braced
   (B) Supine with arms comfortably at his side
   (C) Laying on his left side
   (D) Standing

4. A 35-year-old accountant presents to your clinic for a routine checkup. He has no complaints. He has hypertension, but his blood pressure is normal with medication. He has a normal physical examination. His temperature is 102°F. What is the most likely explanation for his elevated temperature?
   (A) He is septic.
   (B) He drank a cup of hot coffee just before having his temperature taken.
   (C) He has cancer.
   (D) He has hypothyroidism.

5. All of the following areas of the body are used to obtain a temperature reading EXCEPT the:
   (A) Mouth
   (B) Rectum
   (C) Ear
   (D) Umbilicus

■ Matching

Match each numbered item with the appropriate lettered phrase or phrases.

_____ 1. Truncal fat

_____ 2. Long limbs in proportion to the trunk

_____ 3. Generalized fat

_____ 4. Very short stature

_____ 5. Exaggerated stare

_____ 6. Masked facies

(A) Marfan's syndrome

(B) Obesity

(C) Hyperthyroidism

(D) Parkinsonism

(E) Cushing's syndrome

(F) Turner's syndrome

CHAPTER 2

The Skin, Hair, and Nails

■ Case Study: Rash

CHIEF COMPLAINT: "I have a rash on my face that won't go away."

History of Present Illness:
Mary is a 35-year-old electrical engineer who presents to the office for evaluation of a rash on her face that has been present for 1 week. She denies new soaps, detergents, lotions, environmental exposures, medications, and foods. The rash is across her face and the bridge of her nose. She states that she first noticed it after spending a week hiking and camping in the Appalachians. The lesions itch and are painful. She has not tried anything to make it better, but she has noticed that going outdoors makes it worse. She denies any spread of the rash to other areas. She has never had this rash before.

She has noticed some increased fatigue, fever, and weight loss. She denies headache, sore throat, ear pain, nasal or sinus congestion, chest pain, shortness of breath, cough, abdominal pain, pain with urination, constipation, or diarrhea. She does have mouth soreness. She has noticed some increased muscle aches and pains, which are worse in the hand and wrist. She denies early morning joint stiffness or difficulty with being able to move in the morning. She denies temperature intolerance, polyuria, polydipsia, or polyphagia.

She had a tonsillectomy at age 9 for chronic strep throat infections. She has been healthy as an adult. She has never had children. She has never been hospitalized for any reason.

Her family history is significant for a mother with rheumatoid arthritis. Her father is healthy.

She does not smoke; she drinks a glass of wine nearly every night with her dinner; she denies illicit drug use. She completed a master's degree in engineering. She has lived with her boyfriend for the past 5 years.

What parts of the exam would you like to perform? (Circle the appropriate areas.)

General Survey	Breasts and Axillae
Vital Signs	Female Genitalia
Skin	Male Genitalia
Head and Neck	Anus, Rectum, and Prostate
Thorax and Lungs	Peripheral Vascular/Extremities
Cardiovascular	Musculoskeletal
Abdomen	Nervous System

What physical findings are you looking for to help determine the diagnosis?

These are the actual findings on physical examination:

General Survey   Patient is an alert young woman, sitting comfortably on the examination table

Vital Signs   BP 112/66 mm Hg; HR 62 bpm and regular; respiratory rate 12 breaths/min; temperature 100.3°F

Skin   Several erythematous plaques scattered over the cheeks and the bridge of the nose, sparing the nasolabial folds

HEENT   Normocephalic, atraumatic

Sclera white, conjunctivae clear; pupils constrict from 4 mm to 2 mm and are equal, round, and reactive to light and accommodation

Oropharynx moist with erythema in the posterior pharyngeal wall; no exudates; shallow ulcers in the buccal mucosa bilaterally

Neck supple without cervical lymphadenopathy or thyromegaly

Musculoskeletal   Full range of motion; no swelling or deformity; muscles with normal bulk and tone

Based on this information, what is your differential diagnosis?

1. _____

2. _____

3. _____

■ Case Study: Change In Mole

CHIEF COMPLAINT: "One of the moles on my face is changing."

History of Present Illness:
Mr. C., a 62-year-old farmer, comes to your office to have you look at a change in a mole on his face. He just noticed the change 2 weeks ago. He says that the mole doesn't itch, but it has grown larger daily and is darkening. He has not noticed any discharge from the site. He denies being bitten by any insects. Although he works outdoors daily, he does not use sunscreen.

Mr. C. has smoked one cigar daily for the past 35 years. On average, he drinks three beers daily and has done so for the past 40 years. He had a broken tibia repaired 2 years ago.

His father died of complications of melanoma. His mother died of lung cancer.

What parts of the exam would you like to perform? (Circle the appropriate areas.)

General Survey   Breasts and Axillae

Vital Signs   Female Genitalia

Skin   Male Genitalia

Head and Neck   Anus, Rectum, and Prostate

Thorax and Lungs   Peripheral Vascular/Extremities

Cardiovascular   Musculoskeletal

Abdomen   Nervous System

What physical findings are you looking for to help determine the diagnosis?

These are the actual findings on physical examination:

General Survey	Alert older man, resting comfortably on the examining table
Vital Signs	BP 110/60 mm Hg; HR 86 bpm and regular; respiratory rate 24 breaths/min; temperature 98.6°F
Skin	1-cm, black, irregularly shaped, slightly elevated lesion on the right forehead; multiple nevi scattered on the back, abdomen, arms, and legs; numerous capillary hemangiomas on the abdomen
HEENT	Normocephalic, atraumatic
	Pupils equal, round, and reactive to light and accommodation; constrict from 6 mm to 3 mm
	Disc margins sharp; fundi without hemorrhages or exudates
	External ear canals patent; tympanic membranes with good cone of light
	Oral mucosa pink; dentition good; pharynx without exudates
Neck	Supple, without thyromegaly; no lymphadenopathy
Thorax and Lungs	Thorax symmetric
	Lungs resonant; breath sounds vesicular

Based on this information, what is your differential diagnosis?

1. _____

2. _____

3. _____

■ Multiple Choice

Choose the single best answer.

1. A 62-year-old school principal with a history of chronic obstructive pulmonary disease (COPD) presents to the emergency room for evaluation of shortness of breath. You note that his lips, oral mucosa, and tongue are blue. You diagnose a COPD exacerbation. The discoloration of his lips, oral mucosa, and tongue is referred to as:

   (A) Central cyanosis

   (B) Peripheral cyanosis

   (C) Jaundice

   (D) Carotenemia

2. A 30-year-old janitor presents to your clinic for evaluation of increasing weight. He drinks a fifth of vodka daily. He has used intravenous drugs in the past but is now "clean." His sclerae and skin have a yellowish tinge. He has a large abdominal girth. You diagnose him with liver dysfunction. What is the discoloration of his skin called?

   (A) Central cyanosis

   (B) Peripheral cyanosis

   (C) Jaundice

   (D) Carotenemia

3. A 72-year-old retired secretary is brought to the clinic by her daughter. The daughter is concerned because her mother seems to be more confused; she has gained more weight, but her appetite has decreased, and she seems to be more "swollen" in general. You obtain blood tests and diagnose her with profound hypothyroidism. On examination of the skin, you would expect it to feel:

(A) Cool

(B) Hot

(C) Warm

(D) Dry

4. A 42-year-old receptionist presents to your office for evaluation of multiple moles (nevi). She used to sunbathe a lot when she was younger and went to tanning salons regularly until 2 years ago. You are educating her about melanoma. When evaluating a mole, all of the following characteristics are important to note EXCEPT:

(A) Asymmetry

(B) Irregular borders

(C) Color variation

(D) Diameter smaller than 6 mm

(E) Elevation

5. A 52-year-old office worker presents to your office for evaluation of a bump on his face. It appeared 1 month ago and is growing. He denies fever, chills, or itching. Physical examination reveals a 0.4-cm nodule with a depressed center and a firm, elevated border that is flesh-colored. Based on this information, what is your most likely diagnosis?

(A) Basal cell carcinoma

(B) Squamous cell carcinoma

(C) Melanoma

(D) Actinic keratosis

■ Matching

Match each numbered item with the appropriate lettered phrase or phrases.

_____ 1. Macule

_____ 2. Papule

_____ 3. Vesicle

_____ 4. Basal cell carcinoma

_____ 5. Squamous cell carcinoma

_____ 6. Spider angioma

(A) Circumscribed superficial elevation up to 0.5 cm in diameter; filled with serous fluid

(B) Small spot

(C) Initially translucent nodule; spreads; leaves a depressed center with a firm elevated border

(D) Palpable elevated mass up to 0.5 cm in diameter; solid

(E) Fiery red; central body surrounded by erythema and radiating legs

(F) May develop in conjunction with an actinic keratosis; firm, red

CHAPTER 3

The Head and Neck

■ Case Study: Red and Burning Eyes

CHIEF COMPLAINT: "My eye is red and burning."

History of Present Illness:
Mr. E. is a 55-year-old machinist who comes to your office complaining of pain in his right eye for the past 24 hours. He describes the pain as severe, aching, and deep; he has noticed a decline in his vision. He does not wear corrective lenses. He denies any work-related exposures. He denies any upper respiratory infection or allergies. He has a history of hypertension and sees his physician regularly for checkups; he has been told that his blood pressure is controlled by his medication. He has not experienced nausea, vomiting, diaphoresis, or abdominal pain.

Mr. E. has smoked three packs of cigarettes daily for 40 years. He has never had surgery.

What parts of the exam would you like to perform? (Circle the appropriate areas.)

General Survey	Breasts and Axillae
Vital Signs	Female Genitalia
Skin	Male Genitalia
Head and Neck	Anus, Rectum, and Prostate
Thorax and Lungs	Peripheral Vascular/Extremities
Cardiovascular	Musculoskeletal
Abdomen	Nervous System

What physical findings are you looking for to help determine the diagnosis?

These are the actual findings on physical examination:

General Survey	Alert, muscular, middle-aged man, sitting on the examining table, holding his head in moderate discomfort
Vital Signs	BP 160/95 mm Hg; HR 90 bpm and regular; respiratory rate 12 breaths/min; temperature 98.4°F
Skin	No rash; nails without clubbing or cyanosis
HEENT	Normocephalic, atraumatic
	Visual acuity is measured at 20/100 in the right eye (O.D.) and 20/20 in the left eye (O.S.); the right pupil is dilated and fixed; the cornea appears cloudy; the right fundus is difficult to visualize
	External ear canals patent, tympanic membranes with good cone of light
	Sinuses nontender
	Oral mucosa pink; dentition good; pharynx without exudates
Neck	Supple, without thyromegaly; no cervical or supraclavicular adenopathy
Thorax and Lungs	Thorax symmetric, with increased AP diameter and slight hyperresonance over both lung fields
	Breath sounds resonant; no wheezes or rhonchi
Cardiovascular	JVP 6 cm above right atrium; carotid upstrokes brisk, without bruits
	PMI tapping and nondisplaced
	Good S1, S2; no S3 , S4; no murmurs, rubs, or clicks

Based on this information, what is your differential diagnosis?

1. _____

2. _____

3. _____

■ Case Study: Ear Pain

CHIEF COMPLAINT: "I have an earache."

History of Present Illness:
Johnny B. is a 15-year-old high school student who comes to the office complaining of an earache that has persisted for the last 3 days. His mother says Johnny's forehead felt hot at home, but she did not have a thermometer to check his temperature. He has a decreased appetite and a runny nose with clear to yellow drainage. He has been sneezing but not coughing. Some of his classmates are sick with similar symptoms.

Johnny is healthy. He has never had surgery, and he does not smoke.

What parts of the exam would you like to perform? (Circle the appropriate areas.)

General Survey	Breasts and Axillae
Vital Signs	Female Genitalia
Skin	Male Genitalia
Head and Neck	Anus, Rectum, and Prostate
Thorax and Lungs	Peripheral Vascular/Extremities
Cardiovascular	Musculoskeletal
Abdomen	Nervous System

What physical findings are you looking for to help determine the diagnosis?

These are the actual findings on physical examination:

General Survey	Alert, interactive, well-nourished adolescent; appears mildly ill
Vital Signs	BP 100/60 mm Hg; HR 80 bpm and regular; respiratory rate 24 breaths/min; temperature 100.5°F
Skin	No rash
HEENT	Normocephalic, atraumatic
	Pupils equal, round, and reactive to light and accommodation; constrict from 4 mm to 2 mm
	External ear canals patent, with small amount of cerumen bilaterally
	Right tympanic membrane red and bulging; left tympanic membrane dull
	Sinuses nontender
	Nasal mucosa pink
	Oral mucosa pink without enlarged tonsils; pharynx without exudates
Neck	Supple, with shotty anterior cervical adenopathy; no thyromegaly
Thorax and Lungs	Thorax symmetric, with good expansion
	Lungs resonant; breath sounds vesicular
Cardiovascular	Good S1, S2; no S3, S4; no murmurs, rubs, or clicks

Based on this information, what is your differential diagnosis?

1. _____

2. _____

3. _____

■ Case Study: Sore Throat

CHIEF COMPLAINT: "My throat hurts."

History of Present Illness:
Ashley S., a 7-year-old elementary school student, is brought to your office by her mother. She has had a fever and a sore throat for 24 hours. She is normally healthy and has never had any surgery. Other children in her classroom have been sick with similar symptoms. There are no smokers in her household. She has no difficulty swallowing.

On review of systems, you elicit the information that she has had clear nasal drainage and a nonproductive cough. She has not vomited or had diarrhea. Her mother states that Ashley has had a decreased appetite but is drinking liquids.

What parts of the exam would you like to perform? (Circle the appropriate areas.)

General Survey	Breasts and Axillae
Vital Signs	Female Genitalia
Skin	Male Genitalia
Head and Neck	Anus, Rectum, and Prostate
Thorax and Lungs	Peripheral Vascular/Extremities
Cardiovascular	Musculoskeletal
Abdomen	Nervous System

What physical findings are you looking for to help determine the diagnosis?

These are the actual findings on physical examination:

General Survey	Alert and interactive child; appears slightly flushed
Vital Signs	BP 90/60 mm Hg; HR 100 bpm and regular; respiratory rate 20 breaths/min; temperature 103.5°F
Skin	No rash
HEENT	Normocephalic, atraumatic
	Pupils equal, round, and reactive to light and accommodation; constrict from 4 mm to 2 mm
	External ear canals patent; tympanic membranes pearly gray, with good cone of light
	Nasal mucosa pink
	Anterior tonsils increased in size with purulent exudates bilaterally; no evidence of obstruction in the posterior pharyngeal wall; gag reflex intact
Neck	Supple, with no thyromegaly; anterior cervical nodes are enlarged to 2 cm; no stridor
Thorax and Lungs	Thorax symmetric, diameter is appropriate for age
	Breath sounds vesicular
Cardiovascular	Good S1, S2; no S3, S4; no murmurs, rubs, or gallops
Abdomen	Soft, with active bowel sounds; nontender, without hepatosplenomegaly or masses

Based on this information, what is your differential diagnosis?

1. _____

2. _____

3. _____

■ Multiple Choice

Choose the single best answer.

1. A 26-year-old woman presents for evaluation of hair loss. She also has noticed increased weight loss and diarrhea. You diagnose Graves' disease (hyperthyroidism). On physical examination of the hair, what would you expect to find?

   (A) Fine texture

   (B) Coarse texture

   (C) Oily hair

   (D) Dry hair

2. A 25-year-old swim instructor presents to your clinic complaining of an itchy scalp. You diagnose seborrheic dermatitis. What physical findings are most consistent with this diagnosis?

   (A) Erythema of the scalp

   (B) Pustules on the scalp

(C) Dry, flaking areas on the scalp

(D) Ecchymoses on the scalp

3. A 55-year-old construction worker presents to the clinic for evaluation of fatigue and weakness. During the course of the interview, the patient reveals that he has noticed both an increase in his ring size and his shoe size; you ask to look at his driver's license and also at any pictures that he has in his wallet of himself from an earlier time. Upon looking at these pictures, you are able to strongly theorize that he has acromegaly. Which physical finding is most consistent with this diagnosis?

(A) High forehead

(B) Small, recessed jaw

(C) Coarsening of the facial features

(D) Ptosis

4. An 18-year-old college student presents to the clinic with the complaint that her heart is "racing." You obtain blood for thyroid studies and diagnose her with Graves' disease (hyperthyroidism). On physical examination of her eyes, what would you expect to see?

(A) Recession

(B) Protrusion

(C) Clouding of the cornea

(D) Ciliary injection

5. A 75-year-old retired farmer presents to your office for a hospital follow-up visit. He was diagnosed with a stroke and placed on medication. On review of the hospital chart, he was noted to have a stroke in the optic chiasm. What findings do you expect on examination of his visual fields?

(A) Right homonymous hemianopsia

(B) Horizontal defect

(C) Bilateral visual field obliteration

(D) Bitemporal hemianopsia

6. A 57-year-old auto mechanic comes to your office for evaluation of decreased vision in his right eye. You perform a fundoscopic examination and diagnose a cataract. What did you see to make this diagnosis?

(A) Absence of the red reflex

(B) Neovascularization

(C) Hemorrhage in the fundus

(D) Uveitis

7. A 38-year-old warehouse stocker presents to your office complaining of a headache. He has had these headaches intermittently for several years, but they have been increasing in frequency. In your clinic today, his blood pressure is 170/110 mm Hg. His urine dipstick is positive for proteinuria only, and his finger-stick glucose is 100 mg/dL. You diagnose him with uncontrolled hypertension. What finding on fundoscopic examination would support this diagnosis?

(A) Cotton-wool spots

(B) Arteriovenous (AV) nicking

(C) Blurred optic disc margins

(D) Macular star

8. A 50-year-old truck driver presents to your office for a routine physical examination. He denies any medical problems; he has never had surgery; he takes no medications or over-the-counter supplements. He has smoked 1 pack of cigarettes daily for 30 years. He does not use alcohol or illicit drugs. His family history is remarkable for hypertension and stroke. On physical examination, you notice that one pupil is larger than the other by 0.4 mm; everything else is normal. What is the most likely diagnosis?

    (A) Horner's syndrome

    (B) Anisocoria

    (C) Brain tumor

    (D) Tonic pupil

9. A 78-year-old grandmother presents for evaluation of weakness in her face. She has a long-standing history of hypertension that has been under fair control. On physical examination, you note that she has ptosis and miosis of the left eye, and left facial anhydrosis. What is your most likely diagnosis?

    (A) Horner's syndrome

    (B) Anisocoria

    (C) Acute angle-closure glaucoma

    (D) Myasthenia gravis

10. When you look at the tympanic membrane with the otoscope, what normal landmark is present?

    (A) Umbo

    (B) Otoliths

    (C) Stapes

    (D) Tragus

11. A 3-year-old boy is brought to your office by his mother for evaluation of fever, loss of appetite, and emesis. The symptoms have been present for 2 days; the fever is only temporarily relieved with antipyretics. You perform a physical examination and diagnose otitis media. What is your most likely physical finding on otoscopic examination?

    (A) Erythematous, bulging tympanic membrane

    (B) Erythematous, retracted tympanic membrane

    (C) Erythematous, scaly external ear canal

    (D) Erythematous helix

12. A 15-year-old high school student presents to your clinic complaining of pain in his left ear. He noticed that it occurred shortly after starting swimming lessons at the local YMCA. Upon physical examination, you notice that the external canal is swollen and tender during insertion of the speculum. What is your most likely diagnosis?

    (A) Otitis media

    (B) Serous otitis

    (C) Eustachian tube dysfunction

    (D) Otitis externa

13. A 15-year-old member of the high school marching band comes to your office for evaluation of hearing loss. He had multiple ear infections as an infant and

toddler, and he had to have myringotomy tubes inserted in his ears. Additionally, he suffers from many allergies. His hearing is diminished in the right ear. When you place a vibrating tuning fork on the top of his head, the sound lateralizes to the right ear. The name of this test is:

(A) Weber's test

(B) Rinne's test

(C) Whisper test

(D) Romberg test

14. Next, you place a vibrating tuning fork on the teenager's right mastoid process, asking him to let you know when the sound is gone, and then you immediately place that same tuning fork near his right ear. He hears the sound equally in air as against his bone. The name of this test is:

(A) Weber's test

(B) Rinne's test

(C) Whisper test

(D) Romberg test

15. A 22-year-old agricultural worker presents to your office for evaluation of coughing. She has had this cough for 6 weeks; it is nonproductive and worst first thing in the morning. She denies fever, chills, weight loss, or night sweats; she does have clear rhinorrhea and itchy, watery eyes. You diagnose her with allergic rhinoconjunctivitis. On physical examination of the nasal mucosa, what would you expect to find?

(A) Erythematous, ulcerated mucosa

(B) Pale to bluish, boggy mucosa

(C) Pink mucosa

(D) Ulcerated mucosa

16. A 2-week-old infant is brought into your clinic by his parents because they have noticed that their child is having some difficulty with feeding and that there is something strange in his mouth. You diagnose thrush. What is the most likely physical finding you will see upon examination of his mouth?

(A) Koplik's spots

(B) White plaques

(C) Erythematous plaques

(D) Epstein's pearls

17. A 7-year-old elementary school child is brought into the clinic by her mother for evaluation of fever and nausea. Upon further physical examination you diagnose tonsillitis. What are you typically expecting to see on physical examination of the oropharynx?

(A) Exudates on the tonsils

(B) Small tonsils

(C) Hemorrhage of the tonsils

(D) Pseudomembranes

18. A 28-year-old housewife presents to your office for a 6-week-postpartum checkup. She complains of fatigue greater than expected and palpitations. Her hair is falling out as well. She denies sadness or depression symptoms. Before this,

she had not had any medical problems. She is breast-feeding her child and is not on any birth control. She had her first period since giving birth last week. A pregnancy test done in the office is negative. What is your most likely diagnosis?

(A) Thyroiditis

(B) Iron-deficiency anemia

(C) Addison's disease

(D) Sheehan's syndrome

19. When performing posterior palpation of the thyroid gland, you should do all of the following EXCEPT:

(A) Have the patient tip his or her head forward and slightly to the side.

(B) Place your index fingers above the cricoid cartilage.

(C) Palpate between the sternocleidomastoid muscle and the trachea for the lobes of the thyroid.

(D) Move your fingers laterally to palpate for the thyroid lobes.

■ Matching

Match each numbered item with the appropriate lettered phrase or phrases.

EYES

_____ 1. Pupillary reaction to light

_____ 2. Anisocoria

_____ 3. Extraocular movements

_____ 4. Blind spot

_____ 5. Normal visual acuity

(A) CN III (oculomotor), CN IV (trochlear), and CN VI (abducens)

(B) 15 degrees temporal to the line of gaze

(C) CN II (optic) and CN III (oculomotor)

(D) 20/20

(E) Pupillary inequality of less than 0.5 mm

EARS

_____ 6. Weber's test

_____ 7. Rinne's test

_____ 8. Enables optimal examination of adult's tympanic membrane

_____ 9. Enables optimal examination of infant's tympanic membrane

(A) Normally air conduction is two times longer than bone conduction

(B) Lateralization of sound with tuning fork

(C) External ear pulled upward and backward and slightly away from the head

(D) External ear pulled downward and backward and slightly away from the head

NOSE

_____ 10. Turbinates that are visible on inspection

_____ 11. Sinuses that are palpable

(A) Middle turbinate

(B) Superior turbinate

(C) Inferior turbinate

(D) Maxillary sinus

(E) Frontal sinus

(F) Sphenoid sinus

MOUTH AND PHARYNX

_____ 12. Normal number of adult teeth

_____ 13. Raises soft palate

_____ 14. Enables tongue protrusion

(A) 32
(B) 28
(C) 40
(D) CN XII (hypoglossal)
(E) CN X (vagus)
(F) CN VII (facial)
(G) CN VI (abducens)

NECK

_____ 15. Anterior triangle boundaries

_____ 16. Posterior triangle boundaries

_____ 17. Normal position of the trachea

_____ 18. Palpation of the thyroid gland

_____ 19. Enlarged thyroid gland

(A) Sternomastoid muscle, trapezius muscle, clavicle
(B) Mandible, sternomastoid muscle, midline of neck
(C) Presence of a bruit
(D) Above the cricoid cartilage
(E) Below the cricoid cartilage
(F) Midline

CHAPTER 4

The Thorax and Lungs

■ Case Study: Acute Cough, Young Adult

CHIEF COMPLAINT: "I can't breathe."

History of Present Illness:
Mindy is a 29-year-old banker who presents to the emergency room with a 1-day history of progressively worsening shortness of breath. The shortness of breath occurs both at rest and with exertion. She also notes a nonproductive cough that started 5 days prior to the onset of the dyspnea. The cough comes in paroxysms that last for a minimum of 10 minutes and a maximum of 30 minutes. She becomes nauseated and vomits if the paroxysm lasts 30 minutes. She has some fever and chills, but no rhinorrhea, nasal congestion, or sinus congestion. She has some chest discomfort, which she attributes to the persistent cough. The chest discomfort does not radiate.

She has a history of asthma as a child, but it resolved by the time she finished high school. Her last exacerbation was at age 16. She was never hospitalized for the asthma. She is normally healthy. She has two children, both term pregnancies with normal vaginal deliveries. She has never had surgery.

She is divorced and works full-time at a bank to support her children. She is a nonsmoker, rarely drinks alcohol, and has never tried illicit drugs. She has a master's degree in business administration. She does not have time for regular exercise.

Her family history is significant for asthma and hypertension in her father, and hypertension in her mother.

What parts of the exam would you like to perform? (Circle the appropriate areas.)

General Survey	Breasts and Axillae
Vital Signs	Female Genitalia
Skin	Male Genitalia
Head and Neck	Anus, Rectum, and Prostate
Thorax and Lungs	Peripheral Vascular/Extremities
Cardiovascular	Musculoskeletal
Abdomen	Nervous System

What physical findings are you looking for to help determine the diagnosis?

These are the actual findings on physical examination:

General Survey	Patient is an alert young woman, sitting in a chair with her arms folded across the bedside table
Vital Signs	BP 155/85 mm Hg; HR 84 bpm and regular; respiratory rate 30 breaths/min; temperature 99.5°F
HEENT	Normocephalic, atraumatic
	Sclera white, conjunctivae clear
	External ear canals pink; tympanic membranes pearly gray with good cone of light
	Nose patent with pink mucosa
	Oropharynx pink and moist
	Neck supple without adenopathy
Cardiovascular	Good S1, S2; no S3, S4; no murmurs or extra sounds
Thorax and Lungs	Thorax symmetric; hyperresonance to percussion; lungs with diffuse end-expiratory wheezes; no rales or rhonchi; unable to take enough deep breaths to perform descent of diaphragms; decreased respiratory excursion

Based on this information, what is your differential diagnosis?

1. _____

2. _____

3. _____

■ Case Study: Acute Cough, Older Adult

CHIEF COMPLAINT: "I have been coughing and can't stop."

History of Present Illness:
Grant is a 55-year-old farmer who presents for evaluation of cough. The cough has been present for 5 days and is productive of purulent sputum. The cough is worse with exertion but is not improved with rest and can occur at any time during the day or night. He notes shortness of breath and chest pain. He notes loss of appetite; he denies weight loss. He denies fever or chills.

   He had measles, mumps, and chickenpox in childhood. He has high cholesterol and had a heart attack at age 52; he underwent a stent placement at age 52. He had a tonsillectomy at age 5 and an appendectomy at age 8.

   He completed high school and currently lives with his wife and youngest child; they have five children.

   He chews tobacco and drinks two-to-three beers every night. He tried marijuana in high school but denies any current usage.

   His family history is significant for a father who died of coronary artery disease and who had hypertension. His mother is deceased as a result of breast cancer.

What parts of the exam would you like to perform? (Circle the appropriate areas.)

General Survey	Breasts and Axillae
Vital Signs	Female Genitalia
Skin	Male Genitalia
Head and Neck	Anus, Rectum, and Prostate
Thorax and Lungs	Peripheral Vascular/Extremities
Cardiovascular	Musculoskeletal
Abdomen	Nervous System

What physical findings are you looking for to help determine the diagnosis?

These are the actual findings on physical examination:

General Survey	Patient is an alert, ill-appearing older male, sitting upright on the examination table
Vital Signs	BP 132/83 mm Hg; HR 105 bpm and regular; respiratory rate 28 breaths/min; temperature 101.7°F
Skin	No rash
HEENT	Normocephalic, atraumatic
	Sclera white, conjunctivae clear; pupils constrict from 5 mm to 3 mm and are equal, round, and reactive to light and accommodation; fundi with sharp discs
	External ear canals pink; tympanic membranes pearly gray with good cone of light
	Nose patent with pink mucosa
	Oropharynx dry without exudates
	Neck supple without lymphadenopathy or thyromegaly
Cardiovascular	Good S1, S2; no S3, S4; no murmurs or extra sounds
Thorax and Lungs	Thorax symmetric with good respiratory excursion
	Percussion notes are dull over the left base.
	Breath sounds broncho-vesicular in the left base with egophony and E-to-A changes and is diminished; no wheezes, rales, or rhonchi; tactile fremitus decreased on the left side; diaphragms descend 5 cm bilaterally

Based on this information, what is your differential diagnosis?

1. _____

2. _____

3. _____

■ Case Study: Shortness of Breath

CHIEF COMPLAINT: "I have trouble breathing"

History of Present Illness:
Juan is a 57-year-old retired police officer who presents for evaluation of shortness of breath.

The shortness of breath has been going on for several weeks, but it has gotten progressively more frequent over the past week. In the past, it occurred only with strenuous activity, which he has limited. Now, it occurs with minor exertion, such as walking from the front door to his mailbox. The shortness of breath improved with rest, but over the past week, he has had to rest more often. He has a cough productive of yellow mucoid sputum. He denies chest pain, orthopnea, paroxysmal nocturnal dyspnea, and palpitations.

He denies nasal congestion, ear pain, sinus pain, sore throat, neck pain or stiffness, and fever. He has lost 25 pounds over the past 3 months and notes that his appetite is decreased. He denies night sweats. He does not have headache, ear pain, facial pain, sore throat, nasal congestion, or neck pain or stiffness. He denies abdominal pain, diarrhea, constipation, and difficulty with urination. He denies swelling in his legs. He does have some pain in his legs with exertion, but this goes away if he sits down and rests for a few minutes. He denies muscle or joint pain.

He had mumps and chickenpox as a child. He has high blood pressure, for which he takes two medications. He has high cholesterol and takes one medication for it. He had an appendectomy at age 10, a hernia repair at age 18, and an arthroscopy at age 35.

He lives with his wife of 36 years. They have four children. He smokes three packs of cigarettes daily and started smoking at age 15. He drinks a six-pack of beer every weekend. He has never tried illicit drugs. He completed an associate's degree in criminal justice. He used to go jogging but has not had the energy to do this for several months.

His father died of lung cancer at the age of 63. His mother is alive and has high blood pressure; she had a stroke last year and is currently living in a long-term care facility.

What parts of the exam would you like to perform? (Circle the appropriate areas.)

General Survey	Breasts and Axillae
Vital Signs	Female Genitalia
Skin	Male Genitalia
Head and Neck	Anus, Rectum, and Prostate
Thorax and Lungs	Peripheral Vascular/Extremities
Cardiovascular	Musculoskeletal
Abdomen	Nervous System

What physical findings are you looking for to help determine the diagnosis?

These are the actual findings on physical examination:

General Survey	Patient is an alert older male, sitting in a chair with his arms at his side and leaning forward slightly
Vital Signs	BP 135/78 mm Hg; HR 75 bpm and regular; respiratory rate 28 breaths/min; temperature 97.5°F
HEENT	Normocephalic, atraumatic
	Sclera white, conjunctivae clear
	External ear canals pink; tympanic membranes pearly gray with good cone of light
	Nose patent with pink mucosa
	Oropharynx pink and moist
	Neck supple without adenopathy
Cardiovascular	JVP 8 cm above the right atrium; carotid upstrokes brisk without bruits; good S1, S2; no S3, S4; no murmurs or extra sounds; PMI 9 cm lateral to the midsternal line.
Thorax and Lungs	Thorax with increased A-P diameter; hyperresonance to percussion
	Lungs with decreased breath sounds and end-expiratory wheezes; no rales or rhonchi
	Decreased respiratory excursion; diaphragms descend 2 cm bilaterally

Based on this information, what is your differential diagnosis?

1. _____

2. _____

3. _____

■ Case Study: Cough, Chronic

CHIEF COMPLAINT: "I can't stop coughing."

History of Present Illness:

Mr. A. is a 40-year-old high school English teacher who has had a cough for the past 10 days. At onset, the cough was accompanied by a fever. He has coughed up green sputum on occasion, but over the last 2 days, his sputum has become blood-tinged. He has noticed increased shortness of breath with exertion and has had difficulty sleeping at night because of the cough. He has tried using over-the-counter drugs, but these have not relieved his symptoms. He has not traveled anywhere recently. Several of his coworkers are also sick. He denies ear pain, sinus congestion, and sore throat. He has no palpitations, constipation, diarrhea, dysuria, or swelling in his extremities. He does admit to a headache, which has been intermittent for the last 5 days and appears to be relieved somewhat by acetaminophen.

He has smoked two packs of cigarettes per day since the age of 14.

His past medical history is significant for hypertension, for which he is taking medication. In childhood, he had his appendix removed and, later, his tonsils and adenoids.

What parts of the exam would you like to perform? (Circle the appropriate areas.)

General Survey	Breasts and Axillae
Vital Signs	Female Genitalia
Skin	Male Genitalia
Head and Neck	Anus, Rectum, and Prostate
Thorax and Lungs	Peripheral Vascular/Extremities
Cardiovascular	Musculoskeletal
Abdomen	Nervous System

What physical findings are you looking for to help determine the diagnosis?

These are the actual findings on physical examination:

General Survey	Alert, muscular, middle-aged man, breathing comfortably, but appears moderately ill
Vital Signs	BP 150/95 mm Hg; HR 90 bpm and regular; respiratory rate 24 breaths/min; temperature 101.5°F
Skin	No rash; nails without clubbing or cyanosis
HEENT	Normocephalic, atraumatic
	Pupils equal, round, and reactive to light and accommodation; constrict from 5 mm to 3 mm
	Disc margins sharp; fundi without hemorrhages or exudates
	External ear canals patent; tympanic membranes with good cone of light
	Nasal mucosa pink; sinuses nontender
	Oral mucosa pink, without enlarged tonsils; dentition good; pharynx is without exudates
Neck	Supple, without thyromegaly; no cervical or supraclavicular lymphadenopathy
Thorax and Lungs	Symmetric thorax, with increased AP diameter
	Lungs hyperresonant; wheezes in all lung fields; fair air movement
Cardiovascular	JVP 6 cm above right atrium; carotid upstrokes brisk, without bruits
	PMI tapping and nondisplaced
	Good S1, S2; no S3, S4; no murmurs

Based on this information, what is your differential diagnosis?

1. _____

2. _____

3. _____

■ Multiple Choice

Choose the single best answer.

1. A 42-year-old waitress presents to your office for evaluation of shortness of breath. She has had a fever as high as 103°F for the last 3 days and has a cough productive of green sputum. On physical examination, you hear crackles in her lungs. A chest radiograph reveals a consolidation in the left lower lobe. You diagnose her with a lobar pneumonia. When you perform tactile fremitus of the left lower thorax, you would expect fremitus to be:

    (A) Decreased

    (B) Increased

    (C) Unchanged from normal

    (D) Displaced

2. When you percuss this patient's left lower thorax, you would expect the sound to be:
   (A) Dull
   (B) Resonant
   (C) Flat
   (D) Hyperresonant

3. When you perform the test for egophony on this patient, you would expect to hear:
   (A) "EEE"
   (B) "AAY"
   (C) Whispered pectoriloquy
   (D) "OOO"

4. In a patient with lobar pneumonia, you would expect breath sounds on auscultation to reveal:
   (A) Rhonchi
   (B) Egophony
   (C) Decreased resonance
   (D) Increased air movement

5. A 65-year-old smoker presents for evaluation of dyspnea. He has a 100-pack/year history of tobacco use. The dyspnea is exacerbated by exertion. He denies fever or chills; he has not had recent contact with anyone who is sick. You diagnose chronic obstructive pulmonary disease (COPD). On physical examination of the thorax, you would expect to find:
   (A) Increased AP diameter
   (B) Decreased AP diameter
   (C) No change in the AP diameter
   (D) Pectus excavatum

6. Upon auscultation in a patient with COPD, you would expect to hear:
   (A) Stridor
   (B) Delayed expiratory phase
   (C) Late inspiratory crackles
   (D) Pleural rub

7. A 19-year-old college student presents to the emergency room for sudden onset of dyspnea. The general survey reveals that she is 6 feet 2 inches tall and weighs 135 pounds. She denies fever, chills, cough, and sore throat. She is a nonsmoker. You suspect that she has a pneumothorax. What findings would you expect with percussion of the thorax?
   (A) Decreased resonance on the affected side
   (B) Increased resonance (hyperresonance) on the affected side
   (C) Increased resonance on the nonaffected side
   (D) Dullness

8. In a patient with pneumothorax, what findings would you expect with auscultation of the thorax on the affected side?

(A) Wheezes

(B) Rhonchi

(C) Absent breath sounds

(D) Resonance

9. In a healthy adult, the expected measurement of descent of the diaphragm is:

(A) 1 to 2 cm

(B) 5 to 6 cm

(C) 7 to 8 cm

(D) 10 to 12 cm

10. In a healthy adult, the respiratory rate is:

(A) 4 to 14 breaths per minute

(B) 14 to 16 breaths per minute

(C) 14 to 20 breaths per minute

(D) 26 to 40 breaths per minute

■ Matching

Match each numbered item with the appropriate lettered phrase or phrases.

_____ 1. Location, anteriorly, of lower border of lung

_____ 2. Location, posteriorly, of lower border of lung

_____ 3. Trachea bifurcation

_____ 4. Fremitus

_____ 5. Location of bronchovesicular breath sounds

(A) First and second interspaces anteriorly and between the scapulae

(B) Sternal angle anteriorly and T4 spinous process posteriorly

(C) T10 spinous process

(D) Palpable vibrations transmitted through the bronchopulmonary tree to the chest wall when the patient speaks

(E) Sixth rib, midclavicular line and eighth rib, midaxillary line

CHAPTER 5

The Cardiovascular System

■ Case Study: Chest Pain

CHIEF COMPLAINT: "I have pain in my chest and arm."

History of Present Illness:
Mr. F. is a 55-year-old advertising executive who comes to the emergency room complaining of pain in his chest that began 1 hour ago. He describes the pain as pressure under the sternum that radiates into his left arm and up into his jaw. On a scale of 1 to 10, he rates it as a 7 in intensity. He feels short of breath. He has had similar symptoms during the last 2 weeks, but these episodes have lasted for 5 to 10 minutes at the most. He noticed that the symptoms are brought on by climbing the stairs and are relieved with rest. Right now, he reports nausea and sweating. He was given sublingual nitroglycerin by the triage nurse in the emergency room, which has helped to ease the pain.

Mr. F. denies any palpitations, blurred vision, emesis, or leg pain with walking.

He has had hypertension for 25 years and gastroesophageal reflux disease (GERD) for 15 years.

He has smoked one pack of cigarettes per day since the age of 15. He drinks alcohol socially and does not use illicit drugs.

His family history reveals that his father died of an acute myocardial infarction at age 50; his mother, currently living, has hypertension. His paternal grandfather died of an acute myocardial infarction at age 45.

What parts of the exam would you like to perform? (Circle the appropriate areas.)

General Survey   Breasts and Axillae

Vital Signs   Female Genitalia

Skin   Male Genitalia

Head and Neck   Anus, Rectum, and Prostate

Thorax and Lungs   Peripheral Vascular/Extremities

Cardiovascular   Musculoskeletal

Abdomen   Nervous System

What physical findings are you looking for to help determine the diagnosis?

These are the actual findings on physical examination:

General Survey	Alert, obese middle-aged man, who is pale and diaphoretic, with rapid shallow breathing
Vital Signs	BP 160/100 mm Hg in both arms; HR 85 bpm and regular; respiratory rate 28 breaths/min; temperature 98.7°F
Skin	No rash; nails without clubbing or cyanosis
HEENT	Normocephalic, atraumatic
	Pupils equal, round, and reactive to light and accommodation; constrict from 3 mm to 2 mm
	Disc margins sharp; fundi without hemorrhages or exudates; arteriovenous nicking is present
	External ear canals patent; tympanic membranes with good cone of light
	Oral mucosa pink; dentition good; pharynx is without exudates
Neck	Supple, without thyromegaly; no lymphadenopathy
Thorax and Lungs	Thorax symmetric, with good expansion
	Lungs resonant; breath sounds vesicular; no rales, wheezes, or rhonchi
Cardiovascular	JVP 6 cm above right atrium; carotid upstrokes brisk, without bruits
	PMI tapping and nondisplaced
	Good S1, S2; no S3, S4; no murmurs, rubs, or clicks
Peripheral Vascular/ Extremities	No cyanosis, clubbing, or edema; dorsalis pedis and posterior tibial pulses 2+ and symmetrical

Based on this information, what is your differential diagnosis?

1. _____

2. _____

3. _____

■ Case Study: Palpitations

CHIEF COMPLAINT: "My heart keeps beating fast."

History of Present Illness:
April G. is a 19-year-old college student who presents to the Student Health Center because her heart has been beating too fast. This has been happening off and on for the past month; the episodes can occur from one to five times a day and last anywhere from 1 to 10 minutes. The episodes seem to be brought on by walking up stairs and drinking iced tea or caffeinated soda. She denies any association of these episodes with stress. She has limited her activities.

She has not experienced chest pressure, nausea, vomiting, or diaphoresis during the episodes; however, she does feel tired and somewhat lightheaded by the time the palpitations go away.

She is healthy and has no history of other medical or surgical problems.

She does not smoke, drink, or use illicit drugs. She is sexually active but is taking the oral contraceptive pill. She has never been pregnant.

Her parents are in good health, and she is unaware of any medical problems that they may have.

What parts of the exam would you like to perform? (Circle the appropriate areas.)

General Survey	Breasts and Axillae
Vital Signs	Female Genitalia
Skin	Male Genitalia
Head and Neck	Anus, Rectum, and Prostate
Thorax and Lungs	Peripheral Vascular/Extremities
Cardiovascular	Musculoskeletal
Abdomen	Nervous System

What physical findings are you looking for to help determine the diagnosis?

These are the actual findings on physical examination:

General Survey	Alert, thin, young woman, who appears fit and muscular and is sitting comfortably on the examining table
Vital Signs	BP 100/60 mm Hg; HR 65 bpm and regular; respiratory rate 18 breaths/min; temperature 99.0°F
Skin	No rash; nails without clubbing or cyanosis
HEENT	Normocephalic, atraumatic
	Pupils equal, round, and reactive to light and accommodation; constrict from 6 mm to 3 mm
	Disc margins are sharp; fundi without hemorrhages or exudates
	External ear canals patent; tympanic membranes with good cone of light
	Oral mucosa pink; dentition good; pharynx without exudates
Neck	Supple, without thyromegaly; no lymphadenopathy
Thorax and Lungs	Thorax symmetric, with good expansion
	Lungs resonant; breath sounds vesicular with no added sounds
Cardiovascular	JVP 6 cm above right atrium; carotid upstrokes brisk, without bruits
	PMI tapping and nondisplaced
	Good S1, S2 with a midsystolic click best heard at the apex; no S3, S4; no murmurs, gallops, or rubs
Peripheral Vascular/	No edema
Extremities	Dorsalis pedis and posterior tibial pulses 2+ and symmetric

Based on this information, what is your differential diagnosis?

1. _____

2. _____

3. _____

■ Multiple Choice

Choose the single best answer.

1. An 80-year-old woman presents to your clinic for evaluation of palpitations and shortness of breath. You obtain an electrocardiogram, which reveals an irregularly irregular rhythm without discrete P waves. You diagnose her with atrial fibrillation. The most likely physical finding upon auscultation of her heart is:

   (A) An irregularly irregular rhythm

   (B) A rapid regular rhythm

   (C) A midsystolic click

   (D) Bigeminy

2. A 61-year-old hairdresser presents for evaluation of shortness of breath. You examine her jugular venous pulse (JVP) and listen to her heart. You diagnose her with right-sided heart failure. Your JVP measurement is most likely to be:

   (A) 1 cm above the sternal angle

   (B) 3 cm above the sternal angle

   (C) 6 cm above the sternal angle

   (D) 1 cm below the sternal angle

3. A 22-year-old waitress presents to your clinic for evaluation of pain in her chest. She appears to be anxious. The pain is worse with physical exertion, such as climbing stairs. She does not smoke, use alcohol or illicit drugs, or consume excessive amounts of caffeine. You auscultate her heart and diagnose mitral valve prolapse. What did you hear to make this diagnosis?

   (A) An opening snap

   (B) A midsystolic click

   (C) A diastolic rumble

   (D) A holo-systolic murmur

4. What could you ask a patient to do to accentuate the findings of mitral valve prolapse?

   (A) Perform a Valsalva maneuver

   (B) Squat

   (C) Hop on one foot

   (D) Kneel

5. A 75-year-old retired publisher presents to your clinic for a routine checkup. He has a history of class III congestive heart failure, hypertension, and hyperlipidemia. He is doing well and is taking his medications as prescribed. On examination of his cardiovascular system, what would you expect to find?

   (A) PMI in the fifth interspace, midclavicular line, 8 cm lateral to the midsternal line

   (B) PMI in the fifth interspace, anterior axillary line

   (C) PMI in the third interspace, midclavicular line

   (D) PMI in the eighth interspace, anterior axillary line

■ Matching

Match each numbered item with the appropriate lettered phrase or phrases.

HEART SOUNDS

_____ 1. S1

_____ 2. S2

_____ 3. S3

_____ 4. S4

   (A) Occurs during atrial contraction

   (B) Produced by closure of the mitral valve

   (C) Occurs after the mitral valve opens; rapid ventricular filling

   (D) Produced by closure of the aortic valve

MURMURS

_____ 5. Grade VI murmur

_____ 6. Grade I murmur

_____ 7. Grade IV murmur

(A) Loud; may be associated with a thrill

(B) Very faint

(C) May be heard when the stethoscope is entirely off the chest

VALVE DISORDERS

_____ 8. Aortic stenosis

_____ 9. Mitral regurgitation

_____ 10. Mitral valve stenosis

_____ 11. Aortic regurgitation

(A) Mid- to late systolic; opening snap

(B) Early diastolic; decrescendo murmur

(C) Pan-systolic; plateau murmur

(D) Midsystolic; crescendo–decrescendo murmur

LABELING

On the following figure, identify the best places to listen for valvular sounds.

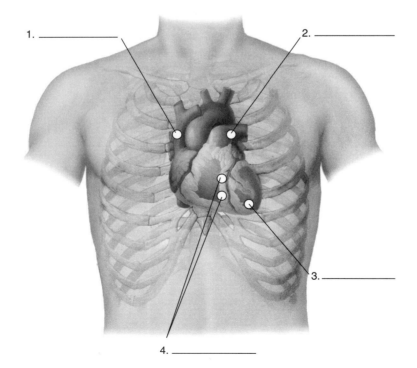

CHAPTER 6

The Breasts and Axillae

■ Case Study: Lump

CHIEF COMPLAINT: "I found a lump in my breast."

History of Present Illness:
Ms. T., a 30-year-old paralegal assistant, comes to the clinic because she has a lump in her right breast. She first noticed it 2 weeks ago. It is tender to touch, and it has decreased in size since her period. There are no changes in the skin over her breast. She denies fever or chills, and she is not breast-feeding.

Her medical history is unremarkable. She has never had surgery.

She does not smoke, drink, or use illicit drugs. She jogs 3 miles daily. She eats a low-fat, low-carbohydrate diet. She is married and has two children, ages 3 and 5.

Her mother had breast cancer at the age of 55.

What parts of the exam would you like to perform? (Circle the appropriate areas.)

General Survey	Breasts and Axillae
Vital Signs	Female Genitalia
Skin	Male Genitalia
Head and Neck	Anus, Rectum, and Prostate
Thorax and Lungs	Peripheral Vascular/Extremities
Cardiovascular	Musculoskeletal
Abdomen	Nervous System

What physical findings are you looking for to help determine the diagnosis?

These are the actual findings on physical examination:

General Survey	Alert, anxious-appearing woman, resting comfortably on the examining table
Vital Signs	BP 128/70 mm Hg; HR 75 bpm and regular; respiratory rate 14 breaths/min; temperature 98.8°F
Skin	Warm and moist
HEENT	Normocephalic, atraumatic
	No occipital, pre-auricular or posterior auricular adenopathy
Neck	Supple, without thyromegaly; no cervical lymphadenopathy
Thorax	Thorax symmetric, with good expansion
Cardiovascular	Good S1, S2; no S3, S4; no murmurs
Breasts and Axillae	Skin without dimpling or retraction; breast contours symmetric
	Nipples without scaling or discharge
	One freely mobile 3-cm round circumscribed lesion, located in the right upper outer quadrant; left breast without masses
	No axillary, infraclavicular, or supraclavicular adenopathy

Based on this information, what is your differential diagnosis?

1. _____

2. _____

3. _____

■ Multiple Choice

Choose the single best answer.

1. A 35-year-old woman makes an appointment at your clinic because she is concerned about a lump she has found in her right breast. It first appeared 3 months ago. It changes with her menstrual cycle and is tender to the touch. She does not have a family history of breast cancer. On physical examination, you inspect the skin, noting the absence of dimpling or retraction. Palpation of the breast reveals a round, 2-cm, freely mobile, tender, circumscribed mass that is firm in consistency and somewhat elastic. The patient has no axillary, supraclavicular, or infraclavicular adenopathy. What is your most likely diagnosis before proceeding with further testing?

   (A) Fibroadenoma

   (B) Cyst

   (C) Breast cancer

   (D) Mastitis

2. A 45-year-old interior decorator presents for an annual exam. In order to examine her breasts, you ask her first to place her arms over her head, and then to place her hands against her hips, and, finally, to lean forward. You notice that her left nipple and areola are retracted while she is in the "leaning forward" position. The appearance of the skin is normal. This finding makes you suspicious for which clinical condition?

(A) Breast cancer

(B) Mastitis

(C) Fibrocystic breast disease

(D) Acanthosis nigricans

■ Matching

Match each numbered item with the appropriate lettered phrase or phrases.

_____ 1. Fibroadenoma

_____ 2. Cyst

_____ 3. Fibrocystic changes

_____ 4. Breast cancer

(A) Soft to firm, round, mobile, often tender

(B) Nodular, ropelike

(C) Irregular, stellate, firm, not clearly delineated from surrounding tissue

(D) Fine, round, mobile, nontender

CHAPTER 7

The Abdomen

■ Case Study: Stomach Pain

CHIEF COMPLAINT: "I have pain in my stomach."

History of Present Illness:
Ms. G. is a 42-year-old housewife who makes an appointment at your clinic because she has been experiencing pain in her upper abdomen for the past 3 months. She describes the pain as an "ache" that sometimes radiates into her right upper back and right shoulder. The pain gets worse after eating fatty or greasy foods, so she has eliminated these foods from her diet. She feels nauseated when the pain occurs and sometimes vomits. She denies fever or chills, weight loss, chest pain, diarrhea, constipation, melena, rectal bleeding, and dysuria. She has not been exposed to anyone who has been sick.

Ms. G. is healthy. She does not smoke, drink, or use illicit drugs.

Her family history is significant for hypertension in her mother and diabetes in her father. Her mother had gallbladder surgery in her mid-40s.

What parts of the exam would you like to perform? (Circle the appropriate areas.)

General Survey	Breasts and Axillae
Vital Signs	Female Genitalia
Skin	Male Genitalia
Head and Neck	Anus, Rectum, and Prostate
Thorax and Lungs	Peripheral Vascular/Extremities
Cardiovascular	Musculoskeletal
Abdomen	Nervous System

What physical findings are you looking for to help determine the diagnosis?

These are the actual findings on physical examination:

General Survey	Alert, obese, middle-aged woman, sitting comfortably on the examining table
Vital Signs	BP 120/80 mm Hg; HR 80 bpm and regular; respiratory rate 16 breaths/min; temperature 99.2°F
Skin	No rash
HEENT	Normocephalic, atraumatic
	Sclerae white, conjunctivae clear
	Pupils equal, round, and reactive to light and accommodation; constrict from 5 mm to 3 mm
Neck	Supple, without thyromegaly; no lymphadenopathy
Thorax and Lungs	Thorax symmetric, with normal AP diameter
	Lungs resonant and clear
Cardiovascular	JVP 6 cm above right atrium; carotid upstrokes brisk, without bruits
	PMI tapping and nondisplaced
	Good S1, S2; no S3, S4; no murmurs
Abdomen	Obese, with active bowel sounds
	Soft, but tender to palpation in the right upper quadrant during inspiration, with a liver span of 9 cm in the right MCL
	Liver edge is smooth and palpable 1 finger-breadth below the RCM
	Spleen is nonpalpable
	No CVA tenderness; no femoral or abdominal bruits

Based on this information, what is your differential diagnosis?

1. _____

2. _____

3. _____

■ Multiple Choice

Choose the single best answer.

1. What is the preferred order for examination of the abdomen?
   (A) Inspection, auscultation, percussion, palpation
   (B) Percussion, auscultation, palpation, inspection
   (C) Auscultation, inspection, palpation, percussion
   (D) Inspection, palpation, auscultation, percussion

2. You are in the emergency room assessing a patient with abdominal pain and fever. You are performing an abdominal examination to assess for peritoneal signs. Which one of the following is NOT a peritoneal sign?

(A) Rebound tenderness

(B) Involuntary guarding

(C) Rigidity of the abdomen

(D) Voluntary guarding

3. A 15-year-old high school student presents to the clinic with a 1-day history of nausea and anorexia. He describes the pain as generalized yesterday, but today it has localized to the right lower quadrant. You palpate the left lower quadrant and the patient experiences pain in the right lower quadrant. What is the name of this sign?

(A) Psoas sign

(B) Obturator sign

(C) Rovsing's sign

(D) Cutaneous hyperesthesia

4. A 25-year-old veterinarian presents to the clinic for evaluation of flank pain, dysuria, nausea, and fever. A urine pregnancy test is negative. A urine dipstick is positive for leukocyte esterase. On physical examination, what would be the most likely sign expected?

(A) Psoas sign

(B) CVA tenderness

(C) Rovsing's sign

(D) Murphy's sign

5. A 40-year-old flight attendant presents to your office for evaluation of abdominal pain. It is worse after eating, especially if she has a meal that is spicy or high in fat. She has tried over-the-counter antacids, but they have not helped the pain. After examining her abdomen, you strongly suspect cholecystitis. Which sign on examination increases your suspicion for this diagnosis?

(A) Psoas sign

(B) Rovsing's sign

(C) Murphy's sign

(D) Grey Turner's sign

6. A 22-year-old celebrity with a known history of intravenous drug use presents to the emergency room for evaluation of a 5-day history of nausea, emesis, and right-upper-quadrant abdominal pain. On general survey, he appears ill and his skin is distinctly yellow. He has a temperature of 102.5°F and a heart rate of 112 bpm. You provisionally diagnose him with acute hepatitis. What would you expect to find on abdominal examination?

(A) Liver edge is tender and 4 to 5 finger-breadths below the RCM

(B) Liver edge is nonpalpable

(C) Liver edge is tender and 1 finger-breadth below the RCM

(D) Liver edge is nontender and 4 to 5 finger-breadths below the RCM

■ Matching

Match each numbered item with the appropriate lettered phrase or phrases.

_____ 1. Liver edge

_____ 2. Spleen edge

_____ 3. Rovsing's sign

_____ 4. Psoas sign

_____ 5. Obturator sign

_____ 6. Cutaneous hyperesthesia

(A) Palpable deep to the left costal margin during inspiration

(B) Palpable 6 cm below the right costal margin in the midclavicular line during inspiration

(C) Pain elicited when the patient's right thigh is flexed at the hip with the knee bent, and the leg is internally rotated at the hip

(D) Examiner's hand is placed on the patient's right knee and the patient is asked to raise his or her right thigh against the examiner's hand

(E) Pain elicited by gently picking up a fold of abdominal skin anteriorly without pinching it

(F) Pain in the right lower quadrant during palpation of the left lower quadrant

■ Labeling

Label the abdominal organs on the anterior view in the following figure.

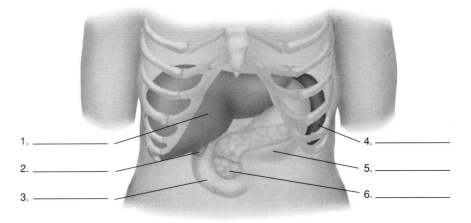

1. _____

2. _____

3. _____

4. _____

5. _____

6. _____

Label the abdominal organs on the posterior view in the following figure.

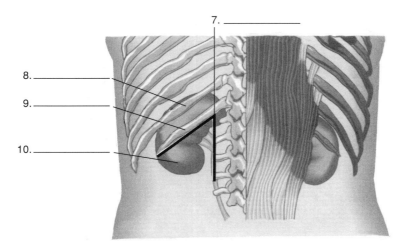

7. _____

8. _____

9. _____

10. _____

Label the arteries on the following figure.

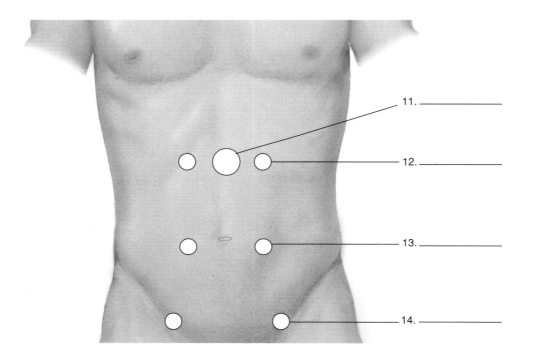

11. _____

12. _____

13. _____

14. _____

CHAPTER 8

Male Genitalia and Hernias

■ Case Study: Urethral Discharge

CHIEF COMPLAINT: "I have a discharge from my penis."

History of Present Illness:
Kevin T., a 20-year-old college student, presents to the Student Health Center because he noticed a yellow-green discharge from his penis the day before. He is sexually active and has been with more than 20 partners in his lifetime so far. His last sexual contact was 3 days ago; he does not know if she had any other partners. He reports no fever or chills; however, he has burning pain with urination and a purulent discharge from his urethra.

He has no medical problems; he has never had surgery.

He is a member of a fraternity and estimates that he drinks at least one case of beer every weekend. He smokes cigarettes and has experimented with marijuana and cocaine, but he denies chronic use of illegal drugs.

What parts of the exam would you like to perform? (Circle the appropriate areas.)

General Survey	Breasts and Axillae
Vital Signs	Female Genitalia
Skin	Male Genitalia
Head and Neck	Anus, Rectum, and Prostate
Thorax and Lungs	Peripheral Vascular/Extremities
Cardiovascular	Musculoskeletal
Abdomen	Nervous System

What physical findings are you looking for to help determine the diagnosis?

These are the actual findings on physical examination:

General Survey	Alert, pleasant, muscular young man, seated comfortably on a chair
Vital Signs	BP 110/60 mm Hg; HR 75 bpm and regular; respiratory rate 16 breaths/min; temperature 98.6°F
Skin	No rash
Abdomen	Scaphoid; bowel sounds active
	Soft and nontender, with liver span 9 cm in the right MCL; edge is smooth and palpable 1 finger-breadth below the RCM
	Spleen is nonpalpable
	No CVA tenderness; no abdominal or femoral bruits; no inguinal adenopathy
Male Genitalia	Testes are descended bilaterally.
	No scrotal or testicular masses, ulcerations, or condylomata
	Purulent yellow discharge present in the urethral meatus
Anus, Rectum, and Prostate	Good sphincter tone; rectal vault without masses, stool is brown and guaiac-negative
	Prostate is smooth and nontender

Based on this information, what is your differential diagnosis?

1. _____

2. _____

3. _____

■ Multiple Choice

Choose the single best answer.

1. A 25-year-old truck driver presents to the emergency room for evaluation of pain in his left groin. He has noticed that the pain increases after lifting several boxes, each weighing more than 100 pounds, to fill up his truck. He has had this pain intermittently over the past 5 years, but it has always gone away on its own. He is here because the pain has not gone away, and he is becoming nauseated. He denies fever, chills, constipation, or diarrhea. He denies urethral discharge; he is married and states that he is faithful to his wife. On physical examination of the left testicular area, you note that there is a bulge when you palpate the inguinal canal as you ask the patient to strain. You listen to the left testicular area and hear bowel sounds. Your most likely diagnosis is:

   (A) Appendicitis

   (B) Testicular torsion

   (C) Hernia

   (D) Pelvic inflammatory disease

2. A 19-year-old college athlete presents to the Student Health Center for evaluation of penile pain. He is sexually active, and his last sexual encounter was 1 week ago. He has had more than five partners in his lifetime to date. You inspect his penis and see a cluster of small vesicles and a few shallow ulcerated areas. Your diagnosis based on this history and physical examination finding is:

(A) Carcinoma of the penis

(B) Venereal wart

(C) Syphilitic chancre

(D) Genital herpes

3. A 15-year-old high school student wishing to join the school's football and basketball teams presents to your office for a sports physical. As part of the physical, you must perform a hernia check. You notice that his right scrotum is markedly larger than his left. He denies pain or tenderness, as well as fever, night sweats, and weight loss. On palpation, you feel a fluid-filled mass in the scrotum but can't get above the mass with your fingers. What is your most likely diagnosis?

(A) Hydrocele

(B) Testicular tumor

(C) Varicocele

(D) Epidermoid inclusion cyst

4. An 18-year-old high school student presents to his family doctor's office for evaluation of acute onset of pain in the left testicle. He has had no problems until this morning. The pain has been intermittent, sharp, and radiates into the left groin. On physical examination, the testicle feels swollen and is tender to palpation. What is your most likely diagnosis?

(A) Epididymitis

(B) Testicular torsion

(C) Acute orchitis

(D) Testicular cancer

■ Matching

Match each numbered item with the appropriate lettered phrase or phrases.

_____ 1. Phimosis	(A) Undescended testicle
_____ 2. Paraphimosis	(B) Ventral displacement of the urethral meatus on the penis
_____ 3. Balanitis	(C) Tight prepuce; once retracted, cannot be returned
_____ 4. Hypospadias	(D) Tight prepuce that cannot be retracted over the glans
_____ 5. Cryptorchidism	(E) Inflammation of the glans

CHAPTER 9

Female Genitalia

■ Case Study: Vaginal Discharge

CHIEF COMPLAINT: "I have a vaginal discharge."

History of Present Illness:
Mrs. M., a 30-year-old dental hygienist, presents to the clinic because of a grayish, foul-smelling vaginal discharge that has been present for 1 week. There is no vaginal itching or burning with urination. Mrs. M. is sexually active in a monogamous relationship with her husband of 10 years. She states that she and her husband have no other sexual partners. She reports no fever, chills, abdominal pain, or pelvic pain. Her last menstrual period was 1½ weeks ago.

Mrs. M.'s medical history is unremarkable; she had a bilateral tubal ligation after the birth of her last child, 3 years ago.

What parts of the exam would you like to perform? (Circle the appropriate areas.)

General Survey	Breasts and Axillae
Vital Signs	Female Genitalia
Skin	Male Genitalia
Head and Neck	Anus, Rectum, and Prostate
Thorax and Lungs	Peripheral Vascular/Extremities
Cardiovascular	Musculoskeletal
Abdomen	Nervous System

What physical findings are you looking for to help determine the diagnosis?

These are the actual findings on physical examination:

General Survey	Alert, pleasant young woman, resting comfortably on the examining table
Vital Signs	BP 112/72 mm Hg; HR 64 bpm and regular; respiratory rate 14 breaths/min; temperature 98.9°F
Skin	No rash
Abdomen	Scaphoid with active bowel sounds
	Soft and nontender, with a liver span of 9 cm in the right MCL
	Liver edge is smooth and palpable 1 finger-breadth below the RCM
	Spleen is nonpalpable
	No CVA tenderness; no abdominal or femoral bruits
Female Genitalia	Vulva and external genitalia are without lesions
	Vaginal mucosa is moist and pink; cervix multiparous, and cervical os is without discharge
	There is a gray discharge in the vault (cultures, KOH, and wet preps obtained)
	Uterus is anteverted, midline, smooth, not enlarged
	No cervical or adnexal tenderness; no adnexal masses

Based on this information, what is your differential diagnosis?

1. _____

2. _____

3. _____

■ Multiple Choice

Choose the single best answer.

1. A 19-year-old sexually active college student presents for evaluation of a vaginal discharge. She has been in a monogamous relationship since becoming sexually active and is married to her partner. She denies that he has been unfaithful. She denies fever or chills. She states that the discharge is thick, white, and curdlike, and although there is no bad odor, she does experience some itching. Upon physical examination of the vagina, you see an inflamed vulva, with a slightly red vaginal mucosa. The discharge is thick and white. There is no cervical motion tenderness. The uterus is normal in size without adnexal masses. Based on this information, what is your most likely diagnosis?

   (A) Bacterial vaginosis

   (B) Trichomonas vaginalis infection

   (C) Candida vaginitis

   (D) Pelvic inflammatory disease

2. A 35-year-old woman presents for evaluation of several new lesions on her vagina. She denies any previous medical problems. She is sexually active. She has had four pregnancies and has given birth to two children. She has had more than ten sexual partners in her lifetime. She is currently divorced but involved in a new relationship with a man whose past sexual history is unknown. On physical examination of the external vagina, you see cauliflower-like lesions scattered on the labia. These are nontender to palpation; the largest is 1 cm in diameter. The remainder of the pelvic examination is unremarkable, and there is no vaginal discharge. Based on this information, what is your most likely diagnosis?

(A) Epidermoid inclusion cysts

(B) Venereal warts

(C) Genital herpes

(D) Syphilitic chancre

3. A 28-year-old housewife presents for an annual checkup. When queried, she mentions that she has noticed bleeding in between her periods for the past several months. She has been pregnant five times and has given birth to five infants. She is sexually active in a monogamous relationship with her husband. On physical examination of the uterus, you palpate an irregular nodule that is approximately 3 cm in diameter. Based on this information, what is your most likely diagnosis?

(A) Leiomyoma or fibroid

(B) Cervical cancer

(C) Uterine cancer

(D) Cystocele

4. A 23-year-old sex worker presents to the emergency room for evaluation of pelvic pain and fever. You obtain a pregnancy test, which is negative. Her last menstrual period was 1 week ago and was normal. You obtain a complete blood count, and the white blood cell count is elevated. On pelvic examination, she has cervical motion tenderness and a right adnexal mass that is larger than 5 cm in diameter and is extremely tender to palpation. What is the most likely cause of this adnexal mass?

(A) Ovarian tumor

(B) Ruptured ovarian cyst

(C) Ruptured tubal pregnancy

(D) Tubo-ovarian abscess

■ Labeling

Label the parts of the external female genitalia on the following diagram.

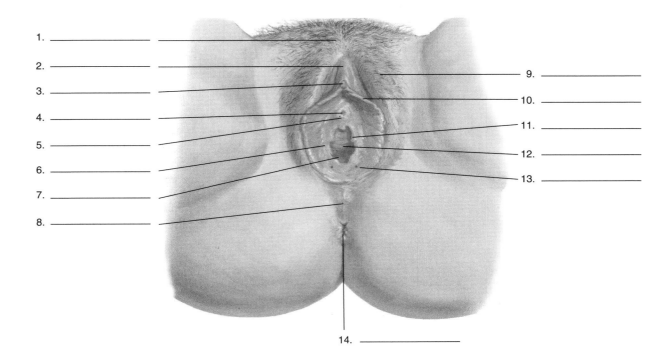

1. _____
2. _____
3. _____
4. _____
5. _____
6. _____
7. _____
8. _____

9. _____
10. _____
11. _____
12. _____
13. _____

14. _____

CHAPTER 10

The Anus, Rectum, and Prostate

■ Case Study: Constipation

CHIEF COMPLAINT: "My bowel movements are less frequent."

History of Present Illness:
Mr. H. is a 75-year-old retired assembly line worker who presents to your office with worsening constipation. He used to have bowel movements daily, but over the last 2 months, the frequency of his bowel movements has changed to one every 3 days and occur only after the use of a laxative. There is no visible blood in his stool, but he does have new hemorrhoids from straining harder. He has tried to increase his intake of water and has added a daily glass of prune juice to his diet.

Mr. H. has lost 30 pounds in the last 3 months and his appetite has decreased. He does not have a fever or night sweats. He does not report chest pain, heartburn, diarrhea, dysuria, swelling in his legs, or leg pain. His activities have decreased due to less energy. Mr. H. has had chronic obstructive pulmonary disease (COPD) for 20 years; the COPD is mild and does not require the use of oxygen at home. In addition, he has had hypertension for the past 30 years and coronary artery disease. He had an acute myocardial infarction at the age of 68. His gallbladder was removed 2 years ago. He had a left inguinal hernia repair as a young adult and an appendectomy during his childhood.

Mr. H. has smoked two packs of cigarettes daily for the past 60 years. He drinks two beers at night and has never tried illicit drugs.

He does not remember the causes of his parents' deaths.

What parts of the exam would you like to perform? (Circle the appropriate areas.)

General Survey	Breasts and Axillae
Vital Signs	Female Genitalia
Skin	Male Genitalia
Head and Neck	Anus, Rectum, and Prostate
Thorax and Lungs	Peripheral Vascular/Extremities
Cardiovascular	Musculoskeletal
Abdomen	Nervous System

What physical findings are you looking for to help determine the diagnosis?

These are the actual findings on physical examination:

General Survey	Alert, thin, elderly man, sitting comfortably on the examining table
Vital Signs	BP 110/75 mm Hg; HR 100 bpm and regular; respiratory rate 18 breaths/min; temperature 97.6°F
	Height: 5'8"; weight: 125 lbs
Skin	No rash
HEENT	Normocephalic, atraumatic
	Pupils equal, round, and reactive to light and accommodation; constrict from 5 mm to 2 mm
	Disc margins sharp, fundi without hemorrhages or exudates
	External ear canals patent; tympanic membranes with good cone of light
	Oral mucosa pink, without enlarged tonsils; dentition good; pharynx without exudates
Neck	Supple, without thyromegaly; no lymphadenopathy
Thorax and Lungs	Thorax with increased AP diameter and decreased expansion
	Lungs with distant breath sounds and delayed expiratory phase; no wheezes, rales, or rhonchi
Cardiovascular	JVP 6 cm above right atrium; carotid upstrokes brisk, without bruits
	PMI nonpalpable
	Distant S1, S2; no S3, S4; no murmurs, rubs, or clicks
Abdomen	Scaphoid
	Soft and nontender, with a liver span of 12 cm in the right MCL
	Liver edge is smooth and palpable 3 finger-breadths below the RCM
	Spleen is nonpalpable
	Fullness in the left lower quadrant, nontender
	No CVA tenderness; no femoral or abdominal bruits
Anus, Rectum, and Prostate	External hemorrhoid at 8 o'clock
	Good sphincter tone; large 1-cm × 2-cm mass 2 cm into the rectal vault
	Stool is brown and guaiac-positive*
	Prostate gland is not readily palpable due to the presence of the mass

---

*Note: Guaiac is a color reagent that is impregnated into filter paper. A stool guaiac test enables detection of blood in the stool that may not be visible to the naked eye. When a sample of stool is smeared on the guaiac-impregnated filter paper and a developing solution is applied, the paper will turn blue if blood is present in the stool. There are a few things that can cause the test to be falsely positive (i.e., the paper turns blue, but there is no blood present in the stool), such as the recent ingestion of uncooked meat, plant material, or large doses of vitamin C (more than 500 mg per day).

Based on this information, what is your differential diagnosis?

1. _____

2. _____

3. _____

■ Case Study: Rectal Bleeding, Older Adult

CHIEF COMPLAINT: "I have been bleeding from the rectum."

History of Present Illness:
Mr. P., a 65-year-old retired farmer, comes to your office because he is worried about a sudden loss of dark red blood from the rectum. He normally has a bowel movement every other day; he does not need to strain. He drinks prune juice daily to keep his bowel movements regular. He reports no fever, chills, night sweats, weight loss, abdominal pain, tarry black stools, or rectal pain. He does feel weak and tired.

Mr. P. has had hypertension for 30 years, well controlled with medications.

He had a left inguinal hernia repair when he was 30 years old.

He has smoked three packs of cigarettes daily since the age of 15. He does not drink alcohol, and he has never used illicit drugs.

His mother died at age 60 of complications of colon cancer. His father had hypertension and died of a heart attack at age 85.

What parts of the exam would you like to perform? (Circle the appropriate areas.)

General Survey	Breasts and Axillae
Vital Signs	Female Genitalia
Skin	Male Genitalia
Head and Neck	Anus, Rectum, and Prostate
Thorax and Lungs	Peripheral Vascular/Extremities
Cardiovascular	Musculoskeletal
Abdomen	Nervous System

What physical findings are you looking for to help determine the diagnosis?

These are the actual findings on physical examination:

General Survey	Alert, pale older man, resting comfortably on the examining table
Vital Signs	BP 90/60 mm Hg; HR 120 bpm and regular; respiratory rate 24 breaths/min; temperature 98.6°F
Skin	No rash
HEENT	Normocephalic, atraumatic
	Pupils equal, round, and reactive to light and accommodation; constrict from 5 mm to 2 mm
	Disc margins sharp, fundi without hemorrhages or exudates
	External ear canals patent; tympanic membranes with good cone of light
	Oral mucosa pink; dentition good; pharynx without exudates
Neck	Supple, without thyromegaly; no lymphadenopathy
Thorax and Lungs	Thorax symmetric with increased AP diameter
	Lungs are hyperresonant; breath sounds are distant, with no wheezes, rales, or rhonchi.
Cardiovascular	JVP 6 cm above right atrium; carotid upstrokes brisk, without bruits
	PMI nonpalpable
	Good S1, S2; no S3, S4; no murmurs, rubs, or clicks
Abdomen	Scaphoid; bowel sounds active
	Soft and nontender, with a liver span of 9 cm in the right MCL
	Liver edge is smooth and palpable 1 finger-breadth below the RCM
	Spleen is nonpalpable
	No CVA tenderness; no abdominal or femoral bruits
Male Genitalia	Testes are descended bilaterally; no palpable masses or hernias
Anus, Rectum, and Prostate	Good sphincter tone, no masses; bright red blood in the vault, no stool to guaiac
	Prostate without nodules
Peripheral Vascular/ Extremities	Calves are supple; extremities are without cyanosis, clubbing, or edema; pedal pulses are 2+ bilaterally
Musculoskeletal	Full range of motion in all joints; no swelling or deformities
Neurologic	Mental status: Patient is oriented to person, place, and time
	Cranial nerves: CN II through XII intact
	Motor: Good bulk and tone; strength is 5/5 throughout
	Cerebellar: RAMs, finger to nose, and heel to shin are intact; gait with normal base

Sensory: Pinprick and light touch are intact and symmetric

Reflexes: 2+ and symmetric, with toes downgoing

Based on this information, what is your differential diagnosis?

1. _____

2. _____

3. _____

■ Case Study: Rectal Bleeding, Young Adult

CHIEF COMPLAINT: "I keep finding blood on the toilet paper when I have a bowel movement."

History of Present Illness:
Mr. S. is a 30-year-old Wall Street trader who comes to the emergency room after noticing blood in the toilet bowl following bowel movements for the past 2 days. He denies pain with defecation. Prior to this, he had noticed increased constipation. He reports no anorexia, weight loss, fever, chills, night sweats, diarrhea, recent travel, or dysuria. He works long hours and is unable to take breaks.

His medical history is unremarkable; he has never had surgery.

He does not smoke, drink alcohol, or use illicit drugs. He does drink six to eight caffeinated beverages daily; he doesn't like to drink water.

His parents are healthy. He reports no family history of colon cancer or inflammatory bowel disease (Crohn's disease or ulcerative colitis).

What parts of the exam would you like to perform? (Circle the appropriate areas.)

General Survey   Breasts and Axillae

Vital Signs   Female Genitalia

Skin   Male Genitalia

Head and Neck   Anus, Rectum, and Prostate

Thorax and Lungs   Peripheral Vascular/Extremities

Cardiovascular   Musculoskeletal

Abdomen   Nervous System

What physical findings are you looking for to help determine the diagnosis?

These are the actual findings on physical examination:

General Survey	Alert, anxious-appearing, fit young man, resting comfortably on the examining table
Vital Signs	BP 115/70 mm Hg; HR 70 bpm and regular; respiratory rate 14 breaths/min; temperature 97.4°F
Skin	No rash
HEENT	Normocephalic, atraumatic
	Pupils equal, round, and reactive to light and accommodation; constrict from 5 mm to 3 mm
	Disc margins sharp; fundi without hemorrhages or exudates
	External ear canals intact; tympanic membranes with good cone of light
	Oral mucosa pink; dentition good; pharynx is without exudates
Neck	No thyromegaly; no lymphadenopathy
Thorax and Lungs	Thorax symmetric, with good expansion
	Lungs resonant; breath sounds vesicular
Cardiovascular	JVP 6 cm above right atrium; carotid upstrokes brisk, without bruits
	PMI tapping and nondisplaced
	Good S1, S2; no S3, S4; no murmurs, rubs, or clicks
Abdomen	Scaphoid, active bowel sounds
	Soft and nontender, with a liver span 9 cm in the right MCL
	Liver edge is smooth and palpable ½ finger-breadth below the RCM
	Spleen is nonpalpable
	No CVA tenderness; no femoral or abdominal bruits
Anus, Rectum, and Prostate	No external hemorrhoids; good sphincter tone; one palpable internal hemorrhoid at 6 o'clock
	Stool in the vault is brown and guaiac-negative

Based on this information, what is your differential diagnosis?

1. _____

2. _____

3. _____

■ Multiple Choice

Choose the single best answer.

1. Which one of the following positions is acceptable for examining the anus and rectum?

   (A) Patient lying down on his or her side on the examining table

   (B) Patient sitting down with arms forward, leaning over the examining table

   (C) Patient standing upright with feet together and arms extended

   (D) Patient sitting upright with arms braced backward

2. As part of a routine checkup, you are examining the prostate of 55-year-old man. He denies nocturia and urinary hesitancy. On physical examination, you palpate the prostate gland and feel a mass. Which one of the following descriptors would you use to characterize this mass?

   (A) Color

   (B) Size

   (C) Presence of discharge

   (D) Presence of rash

3. You are performing a routine physical examination on a 70-year-old retired banker. On examination of the prostate, you palpate a mass that is 1 cm in diameter, hard, and nontender. The patient has had a 6-month history of fatigue. He denies weight loss and night sweats. What is your most likely diagnosis?

   (A) Benign prostatic hyperplasia

   (B) Internal hemorrhoid

   (C) Prostatitis

   (D) Prostate cancer

4. An 18-year-old college student presents to your office for evaluation of rectal bleeding. You obtain a more thorough history and find that the blood was seen when she wiped after having a bowel movement; she has been constipated and has needed to strain to move her bowels. She denies a family history of colon cancer or inflammatory bowel disease. On physical examination, you note a 1-cm, round mass at the 10 o'clock position at the rectum externally. What is your most likely diagnosis?

   (A) External hemorrhoids

   (B) Rectal prolapse

   (C) Uterine prolapse

   (D) Crohn's disease

5. An 80-year-old retired secretary presents to the emergency room because of difficulty having a bowel movement, stating that "it feels like something is coming out." She denies fever or chills and weight loss. She has had constipation and has used an over-the-counter stool softener and increased her water intake. She denies pain with defecation. On physical examination of the anus, you see a doughnut of red tissue, with concentrically circular folds where the anus should be. What is your most likely diagnosis?

   (A) Thrombosed external hemorrhoid

   (B) Anal fissure

(C) Rectal prolapse

(D) Rectal cancer

6. A 24-year-old computer programmer presents to your office for evaluation of pain in the anal region. He is sexually active with the opposite sex. He denies bleeding from the rectum. He denies fever or chills. On physical examination, you note a tender, shallow, ulcerated lesion at the 10 o'clock position on the external anal region. What is your most likely diagnosis?

(A) Human papilloma virus (genital wart)

(B) Syphilis

(C) Herpes

(D) External hemorrhoid

CHAPTER 11

The Peripheral Vascular System

■ Case Study: Leg Pain

CHIEF COMPLAINT: "My legs hurt when I walk."

History of Present Illness:
Mr. V. is a 63-year-old carpenter who comes to the clinic complaining of pain in the calves of both legs. He says that the pain does not radiate into his thighs or buttocks. He does not report losing control of his bowel or bladder function. He has had the pain for 5 years; it gets worse with walking and goes away when he sits down and rests. The pain has worsened from 3/10 to 8/10 over the past 3 weeks.

Mr. V. has a 20-year history of hypercholesterolemia and has been taking medication for the past 10 years. He has a 30-year history of hypertension, treated with medication.

He smoked two packs of cigarettes daily for 45 years, then cut down to one-half pack daily 2 years ago. He drinks three beers per night and denies illicit drug use.

He had a coronary angioplasty 2 years ago. As a young adult, he had an inguinal hernia repair and an appendectomy.

What parts of the exam would you like to perform? (Circle the appropriate areas.)

General Survey	Breasts and Axillae
Vital Signs	Female Genitalia
Skin	Male Genitalia
Head and Neck	Anus, Rectum, and Prostate
Thorax and Lungs	Peripheral Vascular/Extremities
Cardiovascular	Musculoskeletal
Abdomen	Nervous System

What physical findings are you looking for to help determine the diagnosis?

These are the actual findings on physical examination:

General Survey	Alert, obese, older man, resting comfortably on the examining table
Vital Signs	BP 140/92 mm Hg; HR 66 bpm and regular; respiratory rate 14 breaths/min; temperature 98.6°F
Skin	No rash; nails without clubbing or cyanosis
HEENT	Normocephalic, atraumatic
	Sclerae white, conjunctivae clear
	Pupils equal, round, and reactive to light and accommodation; constrict from 4 mm to 2 mm
	Disc margins sharp, fundi without hemorrhages or exudates, AV nicking is present.
	External ear canals patent; tympanic membranes with good cone of light
	Oral mucosa pink; dentition good; pharynx without exudates
Neck	Supple, without thyromegaly; no lymphadenopathy
Thorax and Lungs	Thorax symmetric with increased AP diameter and decreased excursion
	Lungs hyperresonant; breath sounds distant with no wheezes or rhonchi
Cardiovascular	JVP 6 cm above right atrium; carotid upstrokes brisk, without bruits
	PMI is nonpalpable
	Good S1, S2 with a II/VI systolic ejection murmur at the lower left sternal border; no S3, S4; no gallops or rubs
Abdomen	Obese; bowel sounds active
	Soft and nontender, with a liver span of 9 cm in the right MCL
	Liver edge is smooth and palpable 1 finger-breadth below the RCM
	Spleen is nonpalpable
	No CVA tenderness; femoral bruits present bilaterally; abdominal bruit is present; no pulsatile mass is noted.
Peripheral Vascular/ Extremities	Calves are supple
	Extremities are cool to touch without edema
	Radial and brachial pulses are 2+ and symmetric; femoral, popliteal, dorsalis pedis, and posterior tibial pulses are 1+ and symmetric
	Lower extremities with sparse hair; smooth, shiny appearance; and papular erythematous lesions

Based on this information, what is your differential diagnosis?

1. _____

2. _____

3. _____

■ Multiple Choice

Choose the single best answer.

1. A 68-year-old retired kindergarten teacher presents to your office for evaluation of swelling in her right arm. On questioning her further, you discover that she has had a recent mastectomy for right-sided ductal carcinoma in situ. What is your most likely diagnosis?

   (A) Orthostatic edema

   (B) Lymphedema

   (C) Lipedema

   (D) Chronic venous insufficiency

2. You are obtaining an arterial blood gas on the right wrist of a patient in the intensive care unit setting. You perform a physical examination maneuver to assess the patency of the ulnar artery. What is the name of this test?

   (A) Murphy's test

   (B) Phelan's test

   (C) Allen's test

   (D) Obturator test

3. A 55-year-old construction worker presents for evaluation of swelling in his feet. He has smoked two packs of cigarettes daily since the age of 15. He has noticed pain in both legs when walking, which is relieved with resting for 10 minutes. On physical examination, his dorsalis pedis pulses are decreased bilaterally in comparison with his femoral pulses. His feet are cool to the touch when compared with his upper legs. He has no pedal edema. What is your most likely diagnosis?

   (A) Deep venous thrombosis

   (B) Arterial insufficiency

   (C) Venous insufficiency

   (D) Peripheral neuropathy

4. A 62-year-old accountant presents for evaluation of a rash on his lower legs. He has had this rash for several months. He denies fever or chills. The skin itches. He has tried over-the-counter creams without success. He has smoked one-half pack of cigarettes daily for the past 20 years. On physical examination, the skin of his lower legs is hyperpigmented and bluish-red. He has a shallow ulcer on his right medial calf. His dorsalis pedis pulses are 2+ bilaterally, and he has normal hair distribution on his lower legs. These findings are most compatible with which one of the following diagnoses?

   (A) Deep venous thrombosis

   (B) Tinea pedis

(C) Arterial insufficiency

(D) Venous insufficiency

5. A 55-year-old nursing assistant presents to your office because of persistent swelling in her feet. She is a nonsmoker. Her medical history is noncontributory. She has never had any surgeries. She works two 8-hour shifts daily, 6 days weekly. On physical examination, her blood pressure is 110/60 mm Hg; her cardiovascular examination is normal; and her legs have 2+ pitting edema bilaterally without rashes, thickening, or ulceration of the skin. What is your most likely diagnosis?

(A) Orthostatic edema

(B) Lymphedema

(C) Lipedema

(D) Chronic venous insufficiency

■ Matching

Match each numbered item with the appropriate lettered phrase or phrases.

ANATOMY

_____ 1. Superficial veins

_____ 2. Deep veins

_____ 3. Location of arterial pulsations in the legs

_____ 4. Location of arterial pulsations in the arms

_____ 5. Drainage of epitrochlear lymph nodes

_____ 6. Drainage of superficial inguinal lymph nodes

(A) Femoral vein

(B) Femoral artery, popliteal artery, dorsalis pedis artery, posterior tibial artery

(C) Brachial artery, radial artery

(D) Great saphenous vein, small saphenous vein

(E) Superficial portions of the lower abdomen and buttock

(F) Ulnar surface of the forearm and hand, the little and ring fingers, and the adjacent surface of the middle finger

TYPE AND DISTRIBUTION OF EDEMA

_____ 7. Right-sided congestive heart failure

_____ 8. Hypoalbuminemia

_____ 9. Lymphedema

_____ 10. Orthostatic edema

(A) Edema of dependent areas; no cardiac or hepatic signs

(B) Localized edema; involves one or both legs

(C) Dependent edema; sacral edema when patient is supine; may see increased JVP, enlarged liver, and enlarged heart; S3 present

(D) Edema in the loose subcutaneous tissues of the eyelids; may also appear in the feet and legs

CHAPTER 12

The Musculoskeletal System

■ Case Study: Shoulder Pain, Adult

CHIEF COMPLAINT: "My shoulder hurts"

History of Present Illness:
Nancy is a 52-year-old floral designer who presents for evaluation of shoulder pain. She has experienced this pain in the past, but it has always gotten better on its own. Currently, the pain is 8/10. She describes it as an ongoing ache with sharp pain when she tries to reach for objects. It started a few days ago. She has tried over-the-counter analgesics and a heating pad, which helps to reduce the pain for approximately 1–2 hours, but it doesn't relieve it completely. She has been unable to complete her activities as a floral designer, and it is costing her jobs.

She denies trauma or injury to the shoulder in the past. She denies neck pain or stiffness; she denies numbness or tingling in her arms. She has noticed some increased weakness: she is unable to pick up heavy objects and carry them for long time periods like she did in the past. She was healthy as a child; she did break her arm jumping on a trampoline at age 8. She has hypertension and elevated cholesterol, for which she takes medications. She had a cholecystectomy at age 40. She has only been hospitalized for her surgery.

Her family history is significant for a father who had a stroke at age 72; he currently lives at an assisted living facility. Her mother is still alive, and she has hypertension.

She smokes a half a pack of cigarettes daily, since age 15; she does not use alcohol or illicit drugs. She completed an associate's degree in horticulture. She is divorced and lives by herself. She has two children, ages 25 and 28, and five grandchildren. They are all healthy.

What parts of the exam would you like to perform? (Circle the appropriate areas.)

General Survey	Breasts and Axillae
Vital Signs	Female Genitalia
Skin	Male Genitalia
Head and Neck	Anus, Rectum, and Prostate
Thorax and Lungs	Peripheral Vascular/Extremities
Cardiovascular	Musculoskeletal
Abdomen	Nervous System

What physical findings are you looking for to help determine the diagnosis?

These are the actual findings on physical examination:

General Survey	Patient is an alert, middle-aged woman, sitting comfortably on the examination table
Vital Signs	BP 120/82 mm Hg; HR 74 bpm and regular; respiratory rate 14 breaths/min; temperature 98.7°F
Musculoskeletal	Neck with full range of motion; no tenderness to palpation over the spinous processes; trapezius muscles palpated and without spasm
	Shoulder nontender to palpation of the gleno-humeral joint; nontender to palpation in the bicipital groove; decreased shoulder abduction and forward flexion, otherwise full ROM; when the arm is abducted to a 90 degree angle (with the thumb angled downward) and lowered, the arm drops suddenly
	Good muscle bulk and tone

Based on this information, what is your differential diagnosis?

1. _____

2. _____

3. _____

■ Case Study: Knee Pain, Adult

CHIEF COMPLAINT: "My knee hurts and it is swollen."

History of Present Illness:
Cade is a 22-year-old recent college graduate who presents for evaluation of a painful knee.

He first noticed the pain after playing flag football with his friends this past weekend. He denies hearing a pop; he probably twisted and turned to plant his foot, but he can't remember a specific incident that precipitated the knee pain. He has had this pain in the past, and it has resolved with rest and icing of the knee; this time, it hasn't gone away. He has some difficulty with walking and feels that his knee is unstable; however, it has not given way. He does note a clicking sensation when he walks, and his knee has been locking more. He denies any foot drag or drop. He denies any numbness or tingling in his leg.

He is normally healthy. He had a finger dislocation in high school but hasn't had problems with it since. He has never had surgery. He has never been hospitalized. His parents are healthy.

He does not smoke; he drinks a six-pack of beer on the weekends with his friends, usually while watching sports on T.V.; he denies illicit drug use. He is sexually active with his fiancée of 2 years; they plan to get married next year. He is currently looking for work in computer engineering.

What parts of the exam would you like to perform? (Circle the appropriate areas.)

General Survey	Breasts and Axillae
Vital Signs	Female Genitalia
Skin	Male Genitalia
Head and Neck	Anus, Rectum, and Prostate
Thorax and Lungs	Peripheral Vascular/Extremities
Cardiovascular	Musculoskeletal
Abdomen	Nervous System

What physical findings are you looking for to help determine the diagnosis?

These are the actual findings on physical examination:

General Survey	Patient is an alert young man, sitting comfortably on the examination table
Vital Signs	BP 112/70 mm Hg; HR 68 bpm and regular; respiratory rate 16 breaths/min; temperature 98.6°F
Musculoskeletal	Femur, tibia, and patella are in normal alignment when the patient stands and walks; decreased range of motion secondary to swelling and pain; no medial joint line tenderness to palpation.

With the patient laying supine, the knee flexed to 30 degrees, and the femur stabilized, there is a discrete end point noted when the anterior tibia is moved forward (Lachman's test). With the patient supine, the knee flexed to 90 degrees and the femur stabilized, there is a discrete end point noted when the tibia is moved forward (anterior drawer test) and backward (posterior drawer test).

With the patient supine and the examiner's hands on the heel and knee, the knee is extended from a fully flexed position while the tibia is internally and externally rotated (McMurray test). The patient experiences popping with this maneuver as well as an inability to fully extend the knee. With the patient prone and the examiner's knee is placed on the patient's posterior thigh and his or her hand is placed on the patient's ankle, the tibia is flexed and externally rotated, which causes the patient to experience an increase in pain (Apley compression test).

Based on this information, what is your differential diagnosis?

1. _____

2. _____

3. _____

■ Case Study: Neck Pain

CHIEF COMPLAINT: "My neck hurts."

History of Present Illness:
Mrs. O., a 35-year-old data entry operator, comes to the clinic for evaluation of neck pain that has been progressively increasing for the past 2 weeks. She has had neck pain that worsens at the end of the day off and on for 6 months. Two weeks ago, she was in a "fender bender" and was hit from behind. She did not lose consciousness and did not go to the emergency room at the time of the accident. Since then, she has noticed that the pain occurs within 1 hour of awakening and is present all day long. She does not have numbness, tingling, or weakness in her arms and hands. She has not had fever, chills, weight loss, or night sweats.

Mrs. O.'s medical history and surgical history are unremarkable.

She does not smoke, drink alcohol, or use illicit drugs. She is married and has three children. In addition to her daytime job doing data entry, she works as a medical transcriptionist for 4 hours each evening.

Her mother has hypertension and her father, who is a smoker, has emphysema.

What parts of the exam would you like to perform? (Circle the appropriate areas.)

General Survey	Breasts and Axillae
Vital Signs	Female Genitalia
Skin	Male Genitalia
Head and Neck	Anus, Rectum, and Prostate
Thorax and Lungs	Peripheral Vascular/Extremities
Cardiovascular	Musculoskeletal
Abdomen	Nervous System

What physical findings are you looking for to help determine the diagnosis?

These are the actual findings on physical examination:

General Survey	Alert, thin, younger woman, sitting comfortably on the examining table
Vital Signs	BP 112/68 mm Hg; HR 88 bpm and regular; respiratory rate 14 bpm; temperature 98.6°F
Skin	No rash; nails without clubbing or cyanosis
HEENT	Normocephalic, atraumatic
	Pupils equal, round, and reactive to light and accommodation; constrict from 5 mm to 2 mm
	Disc margins sharp; fundi without hemorrhages or exudates
	External ear canals patent; tympanic membranes with good cone of light
	Oral mucosa pink; dentition good; pharynx without exudates
Neck	Supple, without thyromegaly or lymphadenopathy
Musculoskeletal	Diminished range of motion in the cervical spine with flexion and right lateral rotation, secondary to pain
	No vertebral tenderness
	Tenderness over the right trapezius
	Good range of motion in all remaining joints; no evidence of deformities
Neurologic	Mental status: Patient is oriented to person, place, and time
	Cranial nerves: CN II through XII intact
	Motor: Good bulk and tone; strength is 5/5 throughout
	Cerebellar: RAMs, finger to nose, and heel to shin are intact; gait with normal base
	Sensory: Pinprick and light touch are intact and symmetric
	Reflexes: 2+ and symmetric, with toes downgoing

Based on this information, what is your differential diagnosis?

1. _____

2. _____

3. _____

■ Case Study: Low Back Pain

CHIEF COMPLAINT: "My back hurts almost every day."

History of Present Illness:
Ms. Z. is a 28-year-old graduate student in biomedical sciences who has had intermittent low back pain for the past 2 years. Her episodes have recently increased in frequency. She was more physically active in the past but denies any recent injury provoking the pain. The back pain appears to worsen with forward bending and with sitting for long time periods. She has noticed that recently the pain radiates along the back of her right lower leg and limits her activities. She has not lost control of her bowel or bladder function, nor does her foot drag when she walks. She reports no fever, chills, weight loss, or night sweats.

Ms. Z.'s medical and surgical histories are unremarkable.

She takes oral contraceptives and a daily multivitamin; she uses over-the-counter analgesics to relieve her back pain.

Her mother has hypertension, and her father has diabetes.

What parts of the exam would you like to perform? (Circle the appropriate areas.)

General Survey	Breasts and Axillae
Vital Signs	Female Genitalia
Skin	Male Genitalia
Head and Neck	Anus, Rectum, and Prostate
Thorax and Lungs	Peripheral Vascular/Extremities
Cardiovascular	Musculoskeletal
Abdomen	Nervous System

What physical findings are you looking for to help determine the diagnosis?

These are the actual findings on physical examination:

General Survey	Alert young woman, sitting on the examining table in some discomfort
Vital Signs	BP 115/88 mm Hg; HR 72 bpm and regular; respiratory rate 16 breaths/min; temperature 99.1°F
Skin	No rash; nails without cyanosis or clubbing
Neck	Supple, without thyromegaly; no lymphadenopathy
Abdomen	Scaphoid; bowel sounds active
	Abdomen is soft and nontender, with a liver span of 9 cm in the right MCL
	The liver edge is smooth and palpable 1 finger-breadth below the RCM
	Spleen is nonpalpable
	No CVA tenderness; no abdominal or femoral bruits
Peripheral Vascular/ Extremities	Calves supple; extremities without edema; pedal pulses are 2+ bilaterally
Musculoskeletal	Full range of motion in all joints, no joint swelling or deformities
	No vertebral tenderness
	No tenderness over the trochanter or sacroiliac joints
	Good internal and external rotation of both hips
	Radicular pain into the right leg with positive straight leg raise at 50 degrees
Neurologic	Mental status: Patient is oriented to person, place, and time
	Cranial nerves: CN II through XII intact
	Motor: Good bulk and tone; strength in the right gluteals and iliopsoas is 4/5; 5/5 in all other muscle groups
	Cerebellar: RAMs, finger-to-nose, and heel-to-shin are intact
	Sensory: Pinprick is diminished in the posterior right leg; light touch is intact and symmetric throughout.
	Reflexes: 1+ in right knee jerk and ankle jerk, all other reflexes 2+; toes downgoing

Based on this information, what is your differential diagnosis?

1. _____

2. _____

3. _____

■ Multiple Choice

Choose the single best answer.

1. A 29-year-old sales representative for a pharmaceutical company presents to your office for evaluation of pain in her jaw. The pain has been present daily for the past 2 weeks. She denies any history of trauma or injury. Her medical history is unremarkable. She is able to eat without difficulty but hears a clicking sound from her jaw. She denies fever or chills. On physical examination, you palpate the temporomandibular joint and ask the patient to open her mouth. You feel crepitus when she opens and closes the jaw. Based on this information, what is your most likely diagnosis?

    (A) Mandible fracture

    (B) Pterygoid weakness

    (C) Osteomyelitis

    (D) Temporomandibular joint dysfunction

2. A 50-year-old physician presents for evaluation of pain in his right shoulder. The pain has been intermittent for the past 20 years, but over the past 3 weeks, it has been present daily. He has tried over-the-counter analgesics, but they do not relieve the symptoms. Five years ago, he fell on the icy pavement and landed on his shoulder. You perform a physical examination maneuver, because you suspect a rotator cuff tear. What is the name of this test?

    (A) Drop arm test

    (B) McMurray's test

    (C) Anterior drawer test

    (D) Tinel's test

3. A 35-year-old factory worker presents to your office for evaluation of pain in his left arm. He denies any acute trauma or injury. His job involves inspecting jars, and he has to test the opening and closing of the jar lids. He denies fever or chills. On physical examination, there is no swelling over the elbow. You palpate the olecranon process, and he has tenderness on the left lateral epicondyle but not on the medial epicondyle. Based on this information, what is your most likely diagnosis?

    (A) Olecranon bursitis

    (B) Osteoarthritis

    (C) Lateral epicondylitis

    (D) Epicondylar fracture

4. A 27-year-old software specialist presents to your office for evaluation of numbness and pain in his fingers. He has noticed that the numbness increases as the day goes on; at first he noticed it only at the end of the day, but now it is present upon awakening. It is present in both of his hands. The pain started several months ago and is not relieved by over-the-counter analgesics. The patient's family history is significant for hypertension and cerebrovascular disease. On physical examination, his blood pressure is 110/70 mm Hg and his thenar eminence is atrophic. Which tests would you perform to confirm your initial hypothesis of carpal tunnel syndrome?

    (A) Tinel's test

    (B) Anterior drawer test

(C) McMurray's test

(D) Allen test

5. A 35-year-old postal worker presents to your office for evaluation of pain in her joints. She states that the pain is worse in her fingers and wrists; both hands are affected. She notices that it takes her longer than 1 hour to get moving in the morning because she is so stiff. For the past few weeks, she has been having fevers, some as high as 100.5°F. You notice that she has fusiform swelling in her fingers and wrists bilaterally and that the PIP and MCP joints are tender to palpation. Based on the history and physical examination findings, what is your most likely diagnosis?

(A) Osteoarthritis

(B) Rheumatoid arthritis

(C) Gouty arthritis

(D) Ankylosing spondylitis

6. A 55-year-old executive assistant presents to your office for evaluation of pain in her wrist. She states that the pain has been present intermittently for several months, but over the last 2 weeks, it has been present daily. She has taken over-the-counter analgesics for the pain, which seem to help. She denies fever, chills, or rashes. On physical examination, she has pain and tenderness over the right wrist but not the left. She has a hard dorsolateral nodule on the DIP joint of her right middle finger. The MCP joints are normal. What is your most likely diagnosis?

(A) Gouty arthritis

(B) Rheumatoid arthritis

(C) Systemic lupus erythematosus

(D) Osteoarthritis

7. A 13-year-old junior high school student is brought into your office by her mother for evaluation of unequal shoulder height. Her mother first noticed this problem 2 weeks ago. There is no history of birth trauma or recent injury. On physical examination, there is a lateral curvature to the spine. The curvature is more pronounced with forward flexion. Based on this information, what is your most likely diagnosis?

(A) Normal spinal curvature

(B) Kyphosis

(C) Scoliosis

(D) Lumbar lordosis

8. A 90-year-old retired business owner presents to your clinic for evaluation of excruciating back pain. She denies fever or chills. She states that the pain started suddenly but denies trauma or injury to the back. On physical examination, the patient has thoracic kyphosis, which you have noted in the past. You palpate the spine and note exquisite tenderness at L3 and L4. There are no step-offs. The patient has limited range of motion secondary to pain. Deep tendon reflexes are 2+ bilaterally in the lower extremities. The straight leg raise is negative. Based on this information, what is your most likely diagnosis?

(A) Compression fracture

(B) Meningitis

(C) Herniated disc

(D) Spondylolisthesis

9. An 18-year-old college football player comes to your office after sustaining an injury on the field. He states that he planted his foot and had to pivot to catch the ball. He heard a "pop," and his right knee gave way and started to swell. The trainer iced it down. On physical examination, you note increased swelling and tenderness over the right knee. He has significant forward excursion when you perform the Lachman test. He also has more movement of the right tibia when you draw it forward when compared with the left. Based on this information, what is your most likely diagnosis?

(A) Posterior cruciate ligament tear

(B) Anterior cruciate ligament tear

(C) Meniscus tear

(D) Patellar fracture

10. A 23-year-old fast food worker presents to your office for evaluation of pain in his feet, especially the heels. He notes that the pain is most intense when he first awakens, then eases up somewhat after walking for a few minutes. By the end of the day, the pain has returned again to its full intensity. He has tried over-the-counter analgesics without success. He denies fever, chills, trauma, or injury to his feet. On physical examination, he has tenderness upon palpation of the plantar fascia. There are no deformities or joint swelling. What is your most likely diagnosis?

(A) Ankle sprain

(B) Heel spur

(C) Plantar fasciitis

(D) Gout

■ Matching

Match each numbered item with the appropriate lettered phrase or phrases.

_____1. Synovial joint

_____2. Cartilaginous joint

_____3. Fibrous joint

_____4. Spheroidal joint

_____5. Hinge joint

_____6. Condylar joint

(A) Movement of two articulating surfaces

(B) Wide-ranging motion

(C) Slightly movable

(D) Motion in one plane

(E) Immovable

(F) Freely movable

CHAPTER 13

The Nervous System: Mental Status

■ Case Study: Increasing Confusion

CHIEF COMPLAINT: "Nurses report that the patient is increasingly confused."

History of Present Illness:
Mr. X. is a 75-year-old nursing home resident brought to the emergency room for increasing confusion. He has mild dementia and a 1-day history of increasingly agitated and violent behavior. The nursing home reports that he is normally pleasant and easily redirected. He has not had fever, but his appetite has been decreased and he has vomited three times today. He has also had diarrhea for the past 3 days.

Mr. X. has had several lacunar strokes in the past 10 years. He has had hypertension for 40 years and diabetes mellitus for 5 years, but he does not require insulin.

He smoked two packs of cigarettes daily for 50 years, but he quit when he entered the nursing home 5 years ago. He used to drink heavily, but according to his family, he quit 15 years ago. He is a retired factory worker and had work-related exposure to asbestos. His family history is unknown.

What parts of the exam would you like to perform? (Circle the appropriate areas.)

General Survey	Breasts and Axillae
Vital Signs	Female Genitalia
Skin	Male Genitalia
Head and Neck	Anus, Rectum, and Prostate
Thorax and Lungs	Peripheral Vascular/Extremities
Cardiovascular	Musculoskeletal
Abdomen	Nervous System

What physical findings are you looking for to help determine the diagnosis?

These are the actual findings on physical examination:

General Survey	Disoriented, thin elderly man, yelling and moving restlessly on the examining table
Vital Signs	BP 90/60 mm Hg; HR 120 bpm and regular; respiratory rate 16 breaths/min; temperature 96.4°F
Skin	No rash; decreased turgor
HEENT	Normocephalic, atraumatic
	Pupils equal, round, and reactive to light and accommodation; constrict from 5 mm to 2 mm
	Disc margins sharp; fundi without hemorrhages or exudates
	External ear canals patent; tympanic membranes with good cone of light
	Oral mucosa dry; dentition poor; pharynx is without exudates
Neck	Supple, without thyromegaly; no supraclavicular adenopathy
Thorax and Lungs	Thorax with increased AP diameter
	Lungs are hyper-resonant; breath sounds are distant; no rales, wheezes, or rhonchi
Cardiovascular	JVP 4 cm above right atrium; carotid upstrokes brisk, without bruits
	PMI nonpalpable
	Good S1, S2 with a III/VI systolic ejection murmur at the left sternal border; no S3, S4; no rubs or clicks
Abdomen	Scaphoid; bowel sounds active
	Soft and nontender, with a liver span of 9 cm in the right MCL
	Liver edge is smooth and palpable 1 finger-breadth below the RCM
	Spleen is nonpalpable
	No CVA tenderness; no abdominal or femoral bruits
Anus, Rectum, and Prostate	Good sphincter tone, no masses; guaiac-negative, liquid, brown stool in rectal vault
	Prostate smooth and without nodules
Peripheral Vascular/ Extremities	Calves supple without edema; peripheral pulses are 2+ bilaterally
Musculoskeletal	Good range of motion in all joints; no swelling or deformities
Neurologic	Mental status: Patient is not oriented to person, place, or time
	Cranial nerves: CN II through XII intact
	Motor: Good bulk and tone, strength 5/5 throughout
	Cerebellar: Patient unable to perform RAMs, finger-to-nose, or heel-to-shin; patient cannot stand, so unable to assess gait

Sensory: Unable to assess pinprick and light touch

Reflexes: 2+ and symmetric, with toes downgoing

Based on this information, what is your differential diagnosis?

1. _____

2. _____

3. _____

■ Multiple Choice

Choose the best single answer

1. You are evaluating a 22-year-old woman who was brought to the emergency room with an altered level of consciousness. She is drowsy, but she opens her eyes, looks at you, responds to questions, and then falls back asleep. You would describe this level of consciousness as:

   (A) Alert

   (B) Lethargic

   (C) Obtunded

   (D) Comatose

2. You are called to the lock-up unit in the psychiatry ward to interview the newest admission. The patient is speaking loudly and walking quickly but randomly. He states that he is being persecuted by those around him; there is a conspiracy to lock him up and take all of his money because he is the wealthiest man in the world. He has been diagnosed with an acute schizophrenic episode. This type of thought process is called:

   (A) Obsession

   (B) Depersonalization

   (C) Phobia

   (D) Delusion

3. You are assessing a 65-year-old retired lawyer who has been brought into the office by his family for memory loss. You perform a mini-mental status exam to assess his cognitive function. Which of the following is considered a higher cognitive function?

   (A) Calculating ability

   (B) Orientation

   (C) Remote memory

   (D) Recent memory

4. A 70-year-old retired musician is brought to your clinic for a hospital follow-up visit after sustaining a stroke. He is able to articulate words, but they sound slurred or indistinct. You would diagnose him with:

   (A) Dysarthria

   (B) Dysphonia

   (C) Dysphagia

   (D) Aphasia

5. You are evaluating a 55-year-old teacher for altered mental status. You are trying to distinguish between delirium and dementia. All of the following statements are true about delirium EXCEPT:

(A) Delirium has an acute onset.

(B) In delirium, there is always a disturbed level of consciousness.

(C) Orientation is fairly well maintained but becomes impaired in the later stages of illness.

(D) Attention fluctuates

6. You are assessing a patient with mental status changes in the emergency room. You speak to the patient. The patient opens his eyes and looks at you but responds slowly and is somewhat confused. This level of consciousness is called:

(A) Lethargic

(B) Obtunded

(C) Stuporous

(D) Comatose

CHAPTER **14**

The Nervous System: Cranial Nerves, Motor, Sensory, and Reflexes

■ Case Study: Loss of Vision

CHIEF COMPLAINT: "I can't see"

History of Present Illness:

Jessica is a 32-year-old math teacher who presents to the emergency room with a friend for evaluation of sudden decrease of vision in the left eye. She denies any trauma or injury. It started this morning when she woke up and has progressively worsened over the past few hours. She had some blurring of her vision 1 month ago and thinks that may have been related to getting overheated, since it improved when she was able to get in a cool, air-conditioned environment. She has some pain if she tries to move her eye, but none when she just rests. She is also unable to determine colors. She denies tearing or redness or exposure to any chemicals. Nothing has made it better or worse.

She is normally healthy. She had chickenpox at age 10 and a tonsillectomy/adenoidectomy at age 11. She has no medical problems. She has never been hospitalized. She has four children, all spontaneous vaginal deliveries. She completed a bachelor's degree in mathematics and a master's degree in education. She quit smoking 10 years ago (two packs daily for 5 years); she drinks an occasional wine cooler, and she denies illicit drug use.

Her family history is significant for a father with coronary artery disease (he had a stent placed at age 67) and a mother with hypertension.

She denies fever, chills, night sweats, weight loss, fatigue, headache, changes in hearing, sore throat, nasal or sinus congestion, neck pain or stiffness, chest pain or palpitations, shortness of breath or cough, abdominal pain, diarrhea, constipation, dysuria, vaginal discharge, swelling in the legs, polyuria, polydipsia, and polyphagia.

What parts of the exam would you like to perform? (Circle the appropriate areas.)

General Survey	Breasts and Axillae
Vital Signs	Female Genitalia
Skin	Male Genitalia
Head and Neck	Anus, Rectum, and Prostate
Thorax and Lungs	Peripheral Vascular/Extremities
Cardiovascular	Musculoskeletal
Abdomen	Nervous System

What physical findings are you looking for to help determine the diagnosis?

These are the actual findings on physical examination:

General Survey	Patient is an alert young woman, sitting comfortably on the examination table; she appears anxious
Vital Signs	BP 135/85 mm Hg; HR 64 bpm and regular; respiratory rate 16 breaths/min; temperature 98.5°F
Skin	No rash
Eyes	Visual acuity is 20/200 in the left eye and 20/30 in the right eye.
	Sclera white, conjunctivae clear
	Unable to assess visual fields in the left side; visual fields on the right eye are intact
	Pupil response to light is diminished in the left eye and brisk in the right eye
	The optic disc is swollen
Musculoskeletal	Full range of motion; no swelling or deformity
Neurologic	Mental status: Oriented to person, place, and time
	Cranial nerves: I, V, VII, VIII, IX, X, XI, XII intact; horizontal nystagmus is present
	Motor: Muscles with normal bulk and tone
	Cerebellar: Normal finger to nose, negative Romberg
	Sensory: Intact to temperature, vibration, and two-point discrimination in upper and lower extremities
	Reflexes: 2+ and symmetric in biceps, triceps, brachioradialis, patellar, and Achilles tendons; no Babinski

Based on this information, what is your differential diagnosis?

1. _____

2. _____

3. _____

■ Case Study: Dizziness

CHIEF COMPLAINT: "I feel dizzy, and the room is spinning."

History of Present Illness:
Ms. B., a 45-year-old college professor, comes to an urgent care clinic complaining of dizziness that has persisted for the past week. The symptoms started abruptly. She feels like the room is spinning around. The dizziness is worse when she moves from lying down to sitting up. The sensation lasts a few seconds and then goes away, but it causes her to feel nauseated. The first day the symptoms occurred, she vomited. She reports no fever, chills, weight loss, or night sweats. She does recall having an upper respiratory infection 2 weeks before the onset of the dizziness.

Ms. B. has smoked one pack of cigarettes per day since the age of 15. She drinks alcohol at social events. She denies illicit drug use. She is divorced and has two young teenage sons.

She has a history of allergic rhinitis, for which she is currently not taking medications. Her sons were delivered by Caesarean section.

Her mother died in a motor vehicle accident when she was a young child; her father died of a heart attack at the age of 70 and had diabetes.

What parts of the exam would you like to perform? (Circle the appropriate areas.)

General Survey	Breasts and Axillae
Vital Signs	Female Genitalia
Skin	Male Genitalia
Head and Neck	Anus, Rectum, and Prostate
Thorax and Lungs	Peripheral Vascular/Extremities
Cardiovascular	Musculoskeletal
Abdomen	Nervous System

What physical findings are you looking for to help determine the diagnosis?

These are the actual findings on physical examination:

General Survey	Alert, well-groomed, articulate middle-aged woman, sitting comfortably on the examining table
Vital Signs	BP 110/75 mm Hg; HR 65 bpm and regular; respiratory rate 14 breaths/min; temperature 99.3°F
Skin	No rash; nails without cyanosis or clubbing
HEENT	Normocephalic, atraumatic
	Pupils equal, round, and reactive to light and accommodation; constrict from 5 mm to 2 mm
	Disc margins are sharp, fundi without hemorrhages or exudates
	External ear canals patent; tympanic membranes with good cone of light
	Sinuses nontender
	Oral mucosa pink, without enlarged tonsils; dentition good; pharynx has mild erythema, but there are no exudates
Neck	Supple, without thyromegaly; no cervical lymphadenopathy
Thorax and Lungs	Thorax symmetric, with good expansion
	Lungs resonant; breath sounds vesicular
Cardiovascular	JVP 6 cm above right atrium; carotid upstrokes brisk, without bruits
	PMI tapping and nondisplaced
	Good S1, S2; no S3, S4; no murmurs, rubs, or clicks
Abdomen	Scaphoid; bowel sounds active
	Soft and nontender, with a liver span of 9 cm in the right MCL
	Liver edge is smooth and palpable 1 finger-breadth below the RCM
	Spleen is nonpalpable
	No CVA tenderness; no abdominal or femoral bruits
Peripheral Vascular/ Extremities	Calves supple; extremities without edema; pedal pulses are 2+ bilaterally
Musculoskeletal	Full range of motion in all joints, no swelling or deformities
Neurologic	Mental status: Patient is oriented to person, place, and time
	Cranial nerves: CN II through XII intact including extraocular motion
	Motor: Good bulk and tone; strength is 5/5 throughout
	Cerebellar: Nystagmus with leftward gaze; RAMs, finger-to-nose, and heel-to-shin are intact; gait with normal base
	Sensory: Pinprick and light touch are intact and symmetric throughout
	Reflexes: 2+ and symmetric, with toes downgoing

Based on this information, what is your differential diagnosis?

1. _____

2. _____

3. _____

■ Multiple Choice

Choose the single best answer.

1. An 18-year-old college freshman presents to the emergency room for evaluation of fever, headache, and neck stiffness. On physical examination, the patient is resting quietly and has a flushed face. His vital signs are as follows: temperature, 104°F; pulse, 110 bpm; and BP, 105/70 mm Hg. He has no rashes. During the physical examination, you flex the patient's neck and his hips and knees flex in response, indicating meningeal irritation. The name of this positive sign is:

   (A) Kernig's sign

   (B) Brudzinski's sign

   (C) Babinski's sign

   (D) Lachman's sign

2. A 22-year-old daycare worker comes to the clinic for evaluation of fever as high as 103.5°F, headache, and neck pain. She has photophobia and neck stiffness. During the physical examination, you flex the patient's leg at both the hip and the knee and then straighten her knee to elicit meningeal irritation. The patient experiences severe pain. The name of this sign is:

   (A) Kernig's sign

   (B) Brudzinski's sign

   (C) Babinski's sign

   (D) Lachman's sign

3. This is your first day on the medical ICU rotation. One of the patients you have been assigned to follow is comatose. You want to decide whether this patient's coma is due to a metabolic or structural cause; therefore, you examine the patient's pupillary response to light. If the patient were in a coma due to an opiate overdose, you would expect to see which type of reaction?

   (A) Pupils equal and reactive to light, pinpoint

   (B) Pupils fixed and dilated

   (C) Pupils unequal to light

   (D) One pupil fixed and dilated

4. A patient is brought to the emergency room for evaluation of mental status changes. She has a history of a fever as high as 105°F. She has had a headache and symptoms consistent with an upper respiratory infection 2 weeks before the worsening of these symptoms tonight. You are updating this patient's clinical progress. You diagnose her with a coma. You note that her respiratory pattern has become irregular, with Cheyne-Stokes breathing. Her pupils, which were previously equal, are now unequally reactive to light. What is the most likely cause of her coma?

   (A) Drug overdose

   (B) Alcohol intoxication

(C) Uremia

(D) Brain abscess

5. A 25-year-old housewife presents to the urgent care clinic for evaluation of paralysis in her face. She has a history of an upper respiratory infection 2 weeks before the onset of these symptoms. She states that her face is drooping and that she is unable to close her eye. On physical examination, you note that her forehead is smooth on the right side, her palpebral fissure appears widened, and her nasolabial fold appears flattened and she is drooling. Based on this information, what is the most likely diagnosis?

(A) Cortical stroke

(B) Bell's palsy

(C) Horner's syndrome

(D) Stress reaction

6. A 35-year-old reporter presents to your office for evaluation of back pain and weakness in his left leg. He was play-wrestling with his nephew and hurt his back 2 weeks ago. He states that he has noticed tingling in his left leg as well. He has not noticed incontinence of bowel or bladder function. You perform a physical examination and confirm that he is dragging his left foot when he walks and that his Achilles reflex is diminished. You diagnose him with a herniated disc. Which nerve root are you testing with the Achilles reflex?

(A) C5, C6

(B) L2, L3, L4

(C) S1

(D) L4, L5

7. A 75-year-old retired short-order cook presents to the office for evaluation of weakness. He has a history of hypertension; he stopped taking his medication a few months ago because he couldn't tell that it was making a difference and it was too expensive. On physical examination, his blood pressure is 220/110 mm Hg. He has deviation of the tongue to the left side. Which cranial nerve would have to be affected for this finding to be present?

(A) CN I (olfactory)

(B) CN V (trigeminal)

(C) CN VII (facial)

(D) CN XII (hypoglossal)

■ Matching

Match each numbered item with the appropriate lettered phrase or phrases.

TERMINOLOGY

_____ 1. Level of consciousness

_____ 2. Attention

_____ 3. Recent memory

(A) Awareness of who or what the person is in relation to time, place, and people

(B) Ability to retain information over an interval of minutes, hours, or days

_____ 4. Remote memory

_____ 5. Orientation

(C) Ability to retain information over an interval of years

(D) Ability to focus or concentrate over time on one task or activity

(E) Alertness and state of awareness of the environment

CRANIAL NERVES

_____ 6. CN I (olfactory)

_____ 7. CN II (optic)

_____ 8. CN III (oculomotor)

_____ 9. CN IV (trochlear)

_____ 10. CN V (trigeminal)

_____ 11. CN VI (abducens)

_____ 12. CN VII (facial)

_____ 13. CN VIII (vestibulocochlear)

_____ 14. CN IX (glossopharyngeal)

_____ 15. CN X (vagus)

_____ 16. CN XI (accessory)

_____ 17. CN XII (hypoglossal)

(A) Tongue symmetry and position

(B) Pharyngeal movement; sensation on the eardrum, ear canal, pharynx, and posterior tongue

(C) Movement of the palate, pharynx, and larynx

(D) Vision

(E) Downward, inward movement of the eye

(F) Smell

(G) Jaw movement; sensation of the face

(H) Facial movements, including facial expression, eye closure, and mouth closure

(I) Lateral deviation of the eye

(J) Hearing and balance

(K) Visual acuity, visual fields, ocular fundi, pupillary reactions

(L) Shoulder and neck movements

REFLEXES

_____ 18. Ankle reflex

_____ 19. Knee reflex

_____ 20. Brachioradialis

_____ 21. Biceps

_____ 22. Triceps

_____ 23. Lower abdominal reflex

_____ 24. Upper abdominal reflex

_____ 25. Plantar reflex

(A) L2, L3, L4

(B) L5, S1

(C) T8, T9, T10

(D) C3, C4

(E) T10, T11, T12

(F) C5, C6

(G) C6, C7

(H) S1

MUSCLE ACTIONS

_____26. Elbow flexion (biceps)

_____27. Elbow extension (triceps)

_____28. Wrist extension

_____29. Grip strength

_____30. Finger abduction

_____31. Thumb opposition

_____32. Hip flexion (iliopsoas)

_____33. Hip adduction (adductors)

_____34. Hip abduction (gluteus medius and minimus)

_____35. Hip extension (gluteus maximus)

_____36. Knee extension (quadriceps)

_____37. Knee flexion (hamstrings)

_____38. Ankle dorsiflexion

_____39. Ankle plantar flexion

(A) L2, L3, L4

(B) C6, C7, C8, radial nerve

(C) C8, T1, ulnar nerve

(D) C6, C7, C8

(E) C7, C8, T1

(F) C5, C6

(G) C8, T1, median nerve

(H) L4, L5, S1

(I) L4, L5, S1, S2

(J) S1

(K) L4, L5

CHAPTER **15**

Infants Through Adolescents

■ Case Study: Wheezing, Child

CHIEF COMPLAINT: "My baby has been coughing for the past two days, and now he is wheezing."

History of Present Illness:
Miguel is a 30-month-old male who comes to clinic with his mother for evaluation of cough and wheezing. The cough is frequent and nonproductive and is worse at night; he does not appear to be short of breath, however, he has limited his normal physical activities and just wants to sit watching T.V. His appetite is decreased, but he is drinking fluids well. He has no fever. He has a runny nose (clear sputum) and has been tugging at his left ear. He has not had vomiting or diarrhea. He has no sick contacts.

He was born at term via a spontaneous vaginal deliver; his mother had early prenatal care. He has been staying on his growth curve and has been at the normal range for psychomotor development. He has had a lot of upper respiratory infections, but he is in daycare because mom works full-time. His parents do not smoke; they do have a dog in their household.

His family history is significant for asthma in his father when he was a child and chronic allergies in his mother.

What parts of the exam would you like to perform? (Circle the appropriate areas.)

General Survey	Breasts and Axillae
Vital Signs	Female Genitalia
Skin	Male Genitalia
Head and Neck	Anus, Rectum, and Prostate
Thorax and Lungs	Peripheral Vascular/Extremities
Cardiovascular	Musculoskeletal
Abdomen	Nervous System

What physical findings are you looking for to help determine the diagnosis?

These are the actual findings on physical examination:

General Survey	Patient is an alert, interactive toddler who appears to be well hydrated.
Vital Signs	BP not taken; HR 120 bpm and regular; respiratory rate 30 breaths/min; temperature 99.5°F tympanic
Skin	No rash
HEENT	Normocephalic, atraumatic
	Sclera white, conjunctivae clear; pupils constrict from 4 mm to 2 mm and are equal, round, and reactive to light
	External ear canals pink; tympanic membranes dull with retraction bilaterally
	Nose patent with edematous erythematous turbinates and clear mucoid drainage
	Oropharynx moist with erythema in the posterior pharyngeal wall; no exudates
	Neck supple with tender, enlarged (1–2 cm) anterior cervical lymph nodes
Cardiovascular	Good S1, S2; no S3, S4; no murmurs or extra sounds
Lungs	Thorax symmetric; no use of accessory muscles of respiration
	Breath sounds with expiratory wheezes in all lung fields; no rhonchi or rales

Based on this information, what is your differential diagnosis?

1. _____

2. _____

3. _____

CHAPTER 16

The Pregnant Woman*

■ Multiple Choice

Choose the single best answer.

1. A 25-year-old pregnant woman (G1, P0) at 12 weeks' gestation presents to your office for routine prenatal care. When you ask her about how she is feeling, she states that she has been unable to keep down food and that food tastes "funny" to her. You look at her vital signs; she has lost 5 pounds since her previous visit. The fetal heart tones are normal, and the rest of her examination is unremarkable. What step should you take next with this patient?

   (A) You reassure her that pregnancy-related nausea usually lasts only for the first trimester and that most likely her nausea and appetite will improve soon.

   (B) You are concerned about a peptic ulcer and want to start her on medication.

   (C) You are concerned about hyperthyroidism and obtain a thyroid-stimulating hormone (TSH) level.

   (D) You diagnose her with hyperemesis gravidarum and proceed with further diagnostic workup.

2. A 35-year-old pregnant woman (G4, P3) at 24 weeks' gestation presents to your office for routine prenatal care. Her major concern is a backache that began 2 weeks ago and has not gone away. She denies dysuria, fever, and chills but does admit to urinary frequency. She is taking a mild over-the-counter analgesic for the pain and is using a heating pad. You obtain a urinalysis, for which the results are normal. What step should you take next for this patient?

   (A) You give her antibiotics for her pyelonephritis.

   (B) You diagnose her with a kidney stone and ask her to strain her urine and increase her fluid intake.

   (C) You diagnose her with meningitis and admit her to the hospital for treatment with intravenous antibiotics.

   (D) You reassure her that this is a normal part of pregnancy because the hormones are causing relaxation of the joints and ligaments, which changes the normal curvature of the lower spine.

3. A 22-year-old college student presents to your office because she has not menstruated in 3 months. She is sexually active in a monogamous relationship. You perform a physical examination and determine that she is pregnant. What did you see and feel on examination of the cervix and uterus?

---

*As discussed in the authors' preface, no case studies are presented for this chapter because students would need a more advanced knowledge base and more clinical experience to work through such cases or develop differential diagnoses.

(A) Pink cervical os; firm to palpation

(B) Cyanotic cervical os; soft to palpation

(C) Pink cervical os; soft to palpation

(D) Cyanotic cervical os; firm to palpation

4. You are performing a routine examination on a pregnant woman who is at 24 weeks' gestation. She had early prenatal care, no medical problems, and an uncomplicated pregnancy to date. Her last menstrual period (LMP) correlates with the gestational age of her pregnancy. You would expect the following to be true at her 24-week checkup:

(A) The patient will feel the baby move.

(B) The fundal height will be 20 cm.

(C) The fetal heart rate will be 60 bpm.

(D) The uterus will be anteverted and pear-shaped.

5. You are performing a routine checkup on a pregnant woman who is at 37 weeks' gestation. Her blood pressure is 110/65 mm Hg. The size of the uterus is appropriate for her dates; the fetal heart rate is in the 140s. She has trace pedal edema. You perform an examination for the size of the fetus and its position. What is this maneuver called?

(A) Nägele's maneuver

(B) Leopold's maneuvers

(C) Bickley's maneuver

(D) Bates' maneuver

Matching

Match each numbered item with the appropriate lettered phrase or phrases.

_____ 1. EDC

_____ 2. LMP

_____ 3. Nägele's rule

_____ 4. Leopold's maneuvers

(A) Calculation to determine expected date of confinement

(B) Date of delivery

(C) Technique to determine size and position of the fetus

(D) Most recent onset of menses

CHAPTER 17

The Older Adult

■ Case Study: Urinary Incontinence

CHIEF COMPLAINT: "I am losing control of my bladder"

History of Present Illness:
Trudy is a 72-year-old retired preacher's wife who comes to your office and states that losing control of her bladder is embarrassing and that she can't go out "anywhere" because she needs to be close to a bathroom. She had this problem in the past, but never this badly. She denies burning pain with urination, hematuria, incomplete emptying, and urinary hesitancy. The problem is worse with coughing and sneezing. She comes to the office now because she is losing control of her urine on a daily basis instead of one or twice a week, and it seems more urine is leaking out than before. She does not have fever, chills, nausea, or vomiting; she does not have back pain or leg pain, leg numbness, or leg tingling.

She had chickenpox as a child; she had her tonsils and adenoids out as well as her appendix before age 15. She had five children, all spontaneous vaginal deliveries with no complications. She was hospitalized for the birth of her children and when she had her gallbladder and uterus taken out. She takes medication to control heartburn and for osteoarthritis pain. She does not have any chronic medical conditions. She never used tobacco products; she does not drink alcohol; she never used illicit drugs; and she worked alongside her husband in the missionary field.

She denies fatigue, weight loss, night sweats, headache, vision or hearing changes, nasal or sinus congestion, sore throat, neck pain/stiffness, shortness of breath, chest pain, abdominal pain, constipation, diarrhea, polyuria, polydipsia, and polyphagia. She does have pain in her wrists, shoulders, hips, and knees.

What parts of the exam would you like to perform? (Circle the appropriate areas.)

General Survey	Breasts and Axillae
Vital Signs	Female Genitalia
Skin	Male Genitalia
Head and Neck	Anus, Rectum, and Prostate
Thorax and Lungs	Peripheral Vascular/Extremities
Cardiovascular	Musculoskeletal
Abdomen	Nervous System

What physical findings are you looking for to help determine the diagnosis?

These are the actual findings on physical examination:

General Survey	Patient is an alert older woman who appears her stated age, sitting comfortably on the examination table
Vital Signs	BP 110/75 mm Hg; HR 70 bpm and regular; respiratory rate 12 breaths/min; temperature 99.1°F
Abdomen	Soft, nontender to palpation, nondistended; no CVA tenderness
Genitourinary	Normal female external genitalia with a grade II cystocele.
	Vaginal mucosa atrophic; no adnexal masses; rectum with normal sphincter tone; stool in vault is brown and guaiac-negative
Musculoskeletal	Full range of motion; hands with increased thickness in the fingers, no nodules
Neurologic	Mental Status: Alert, oriented to person, place, and time
	Cranial Nerves: CN II through XII intact
	Motor: Good bulk and tone; strength 5/5 in lower extremities
	Cerebellar: Negative Romberg
	Sensory: Intact to pinprick, light touch, vibration in the lower extremities
	Reflexes: Patellar and Achilles 2+ and symmetric with toes downgoing

Based on this information, what is your differential diagnosis?

1. _____

2. _____

3. _____

■ Case Study: Memory Loss

CHIEF COMPLAINT: "I am concerned that my mother seems more forgetful lately."

History of Present Illness:

Mrs. Novello is a 60-year-old attorney who brings in her 82-year-old mother for evaluation. Her mother, Catherine, seems to be more "forgetful." With further questioning, she appears to be losing track of time: she shows up late or on a different day, or she doesn't show up at all. Mrs. Novello has tried to remind her mother by keeping a calendar for her. The patient hasn't attended her weekly bridge night with her friends. She hasn't been answering the telephone for the past week; when her daughter comes over to her house, she states that she didn't hear the telephone ring. Her husband of 65 years died 6 weeks ago. The patient admits to being sad and lonely after the death of her husband, but she doesn't think that she has a problem with her memory. Her daughter notes that when she has come over, the house is messy and her mother is still in her nightgown. Her mother has not bought groceries in the past 4–5 days, and there is no trash visible that at least indicates that she ate. She has stacks of newspapers all over the house, which seem to have accumulated in the past 8 weeks. When her daughter asked if she was hungry, her mother stated, "I ate already."

The patient had measles, mumps, and chickenpox as a child. She has high blood pressure, for which she takes medication; this was diagnosed 35 years ago. She has never had heart problems. She has never had a stroke. She had a hysterectomy at age 48 for increased bleeding. She had her appendix removed at age 9. She had six children, all vaginal deliveries. She completed high school. She worked as a clerk in a grocery store until her first child was born, and then she worked in the home. She lives alone currently. She never smoked and does not drink alcohol.

She denies fever, chills, weight loss, night sweats, insomnia, and fatigue. She denies headache, changes in her hearing or vision, sore throat, cough, chest pain, abdominal pain, constipation, diarrhea, and swelling in her legs. She denies insomnia, anxiety, hearing voices, and seeing things that other people around her don't see. She denies problems with her ability to walk; she has never fallen.

What parts of the exam would you like to perform? (Circle the appropriate areas.)

General Survey	Breasts and Axillae
Vital Signs	Female Genitalia
Skin	Male Genitalia
Head and Neck	Anus, Rectum, and Prostate
Thorax and Lungs	Peripheral Vascular/Extremities
Cardiovascular	Musculoskeletal
Abdomen	Nervous System

What physical findings are you looking for to help determine the diagnosis?

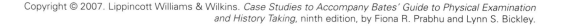

These are the actual findings on physical examination:

General Survey	Patient is an alert elderly woman, sitting comfortably on the examination table with a flat affect.
Vital Signs	BP 160/100 mm Hg; HR 75 bpm and regular; respiratory rate 14 breaths/min; temperature 97.5°F
HEENT	Normocephalic, atraumatic
	Sclera white, conjunctivae clear; pupils constrict from 4 mm to 2 mm and are equal, round, and reactive to light and accommodation; fundi with sharp discs
	External ear canals pink; tympanic membranes pearly gray with good cone of light
Cardiovascular	Good S1, S2; no S3, S4; no murmurs or extra sounds
Neurologic: Mental Status	Appearance: Hair groomed, no make-up; clothes are clean and neatly kept; no increased psychomotor activity with interview. She appears to have difficulty completing a sentence when you ask her a question; she has to think of the word to say.
	Mood: Mildly depressed; affect is flat.
	The patient was asked today's date; she got the day of the week wrong and had to be prompted for the year. She was asked about her current location; she looked to her daughter for the answer. She was asked the current president; she was correct. She was asked to repeat the sentence "No ifs, ands, or buts"; she was able to repeat the sentence back to the interviewer.
	She was asked to repeat three object words and then told that she would be asked to repeat the words back to the examiner after 1 minute; the patient was only able to recall one word.
	She was asked to spell the word *world* backwards and was only able to state "dl"; she spent several minutes trying to think of the next letter out loud. She was asked to subtract 7 from 100, and then from that result, subtract another 7, etc.; she was only able to tell the interviewer the correct answer for the first subtraction.
	Her speech was coherent and logical; no tangents or circumstantiality
Neurologic: Cranial Nerves, Motor, Sensory, and Reflexes	Cranial nerves: CN II-XII intact
	Motor: Good bulk and tone; strength 5/5 throughout
	Cerebellar: Normal finger to nose; negative Romberg
	Sensory: Intact to pinprick and light touch
	Reflexes: 2+ and symmetric throughout; toes upgoing

Based on this information, what is your differential diagnosis?

1. _____

2. _____

3. _____

■ Case Study: Abnormal Gait

CHIEF COMPLAINT: "I am losing my balance when I walk"

History of Present Illness:
Mrs. Gonzales is a 67-year-old retired administrative assistant who presents to your clinic for evaluation of her gait. Her daughter made her come in for a check-up because she was concerned about falls. The patient states that this used to happen occasionally, but now it happens every day. She is not sure about the time frame, but this has been going on for several months, maybe more than a year. She used to walk 2 miles every day since she retired 2 years ago, but she has gradually limited her activities. She denies falling, but she is scared about this. She denies dizziness, headache, tinnitus, visual changes (she is nearsighted and wears corrective lenses), pain in her legs with walking, and numbness and tingling in the feet.

She had the "usual" childhood diseases. She has hypertension and high cholesterol, for which she takes medications. She had a cholecystectomy at age 45. She had four children, all spontaneous vaginal deliveries. She completed high school. She owns her own home, and her youngest daughter, who is between jobs and husbands, lives with her. She quit smoking 10 years ago (forty pack/year history); she does not drink alcohol; she tried marijuana in high school, but it did not become a habit.

Her mother died of a heart attack, and, prior to this, she had osteoporosis and a hip fracture. Her father died of colon cancer. She has two brothers and one sister, all of whom have hypertension. One of her brothers had a heart attack at age 62.

She denies headache, ear pain, eye pain, sore throat, neck pain or stiffness, chest pain, abdominal pain, constipation, diarrhea, dysuria, vaginal discharge, joint pain, and muscle pain. She admits to some generalized fatigue and increased irritability. She has noticed a slight tremor in her hand when she is still, but it goes away when she is actively using her hands, which is most of the time while she is awake.

What parts of the exam would you like to perform? (Circle the appropriate areas.)

General Survey	Breasts and Axillae
Vital Signs	Female Genitalia
Skin	Male Genitalia
Head and Neck	Anus, Rectum, and Prostate
Thorax and Lungs	Peripheral Vascular/Extremities
Cardiovascular	Musculoskeletal
Abdomen	Nervous System

What physical findings are you looking for to help determine the diagnosis?

These are the actual findings on physical examination:

General Survey	Patient is an alert older woman, sitting comfortably on the examination table.
Vital signs	BP 135/82 mm Hg; HR 65 bpm and regular; respiratory rate 18 breaths/min; temperature 97.4°F
HEENT (limited)	Normocephalic, atraumatic; no head tremor
	Visual acuity 20/40 bilaterally; visual fields intact; pupils constrict from 3 mm to 2 mm and are equal, round, and reactive to light
	External ear canals pink; tympanic membranes pearly gray with good cone of light
Cardiovascular	Good S1, S2; no S3, S4; no murmurs or extra sounds
Peripheral Vascular	No cyanosis, clubbing, or edema; no varicosities; dorsalis pedis and posterior tibial pulses 2+ bilaterally
Musculoskeletal	Full range of motion; no swelling or deformity
Neurologic	Cranial nerves: CN VII is impaired: her ability to smile/frown is somewhat diminished; remaining CNs are intact
	Motor: Muscles with normal bulk and tone and no cogwheel rigidity; motor strength 5/5 in upper and lower extremities; resting tremor, 3 cps (cycles per second) in the right hand: thumb and forefinger involved, subtle; negative straight leg raise
	Cerebellar: Negative Romberg
	Sensory: Pinprick, temperature, fine touch intact; vibration reduced on the big toes bilaterally
	Reflexes: Deep tendon reflexes 2/4 in biceps, triceps, patellar, and Achilles tendons; no Babinski
	You ask the patient to rise out of the chair and walk across the room. She needs to push herself up using the arms of her chair and has a slight backward movement to steady her when she starts to walk. She moves more slowly than expected.

Based on this information, what is your differential diagnosis?

1. _____

2. _____

3. _____

■ Multiple Choice

Choose the single best answer

1. Which of the following changes in blood pressure is expected during the process of aging?

    (A) Decrease in systolic BP

    (B) Increase in diastolic BP

    (C) Increase in BP with rising from a sitting to a standing position

    (D) No change in systolic BP

2. A 78-year-old retired teacher presents to the emergency room for evaluation of a fainting spell. He had no warning signs; he just lost consciousness. His wife states that he came around after 1 minute and appeared to know where he was and spoke to her clearly when he opened his eyes. Over the past 3 weeks, he has had similar episodes, where he felt like he was going to faint but hadn't actually fainted. On physical examination, his vital signs are stable. His pulse appears to be irregular but in a clear pattern—there is a pause for every third beat. This is a description of which one of the following conditions?

    (A) Postural hypotension

    (B) Ventricular ectopy

    (C) Isolated systolic hypertension

    (D) Atrial fibrillation

3. A 66-year-old retired waitress presents to the clinic for evaluation of a possible allergy flare-up after the recent changes in weather. She complains of itchy, watery eyes and some increased blurring in her vision. It has been 3 years since her last eye examination. She states that she has had 20/20 vision in the past. You perform a thorough eye examination. Which of the following would you expect to see as part of the aging process?

    (A) No change in visual acuity

    (B) Blurring of near vision

    (C) Blurring of far vision

    (D) Cataracts

4. An 83-year-old retired accountant presents with his wife. She is concerned about his hearing. He denies any problems. She states that he doesn't hear her when she asks him to do something if she forgets to face him as she speaks to him. This has been going on for the past year. Which of the following is the most likely reason for his inability to hear his wife?

    (A) Loss of acuity for high-pitched sounds

    (B) Loss of acuity for middle-range sounds

    (C) Increased acuity for high-pitched sounds

    (D) Increased acuity for middle-range sounds

5. Which of the following abnormal heart sounds/murmurs is more likely to be heard in an older adult population?

    (A) Mitral valve prolapse

    (B) Sinus tachycardia

(C) Aortic stenosis

(D) Aortic regurgitation

6. A 75-year-old retired housewife presents for evaluation of pain with intercourse. She went through menopause (nonsurgical) at the age of 55; she is not taking hormone replacement therapy. What would you expect to see on physical examination of the vagina?

(A) Pale vaginal mucosa

(B) Pink vaginal mucosa

(C) Blue vaginal mucosa

(D) Purple vaginal mucosa

7. A 68-year-old retired hair dresser presents to your office because she is concerned about her memory. She has noticed that she misplaces her keys more often and forgets what she is supposed to buy from the grocery store. She denies getting lost in familiar places; she denies forgetting the names of common objects. She denies being under any unusual stresses and states that her mood has not changed. She has a strong support system and remains active in many volunteer organizations. You perform a mini-mental state examination, and she receives a total score of 26 out of a total of 28. Based on this information, what is your most likely diagnosis?

(A) Benign forgetfulness

(B) Dementia

(C) Meningitis

(D) Depression

8. An 88-year-old retired business manager presents for an annual check-up. He has a history of hypertension. An ECG (electrocardiogram) is obtained as part of the visit. The ECG shows evidence of a prior myocardial infarction. Which of the following symptoms of a heart attack would be typical for his age?

(A) Substernal chest pain

(B) Substernal chest pressure

(C) Shortness of breath

(D) Weight loss

9. Which of the following conditions is considered to be a geriatric syndrome?

(A) Atrial fibrillation

(B) Depression

(C) Falls

(D) Hypertension

10. Which of the following is considered to be activities of daily living?

(A) Shopping

(B) Laundry

(C) Dressing

(D) Food preparation

References

Abnormal Gait

MD Consult. First Consult. Available at: http://www.firstconsult.com/home/us_sands/01220332/senior_adult.htm?id. Accessed April 24, 2005.

Breast Lump

Bickley LS. Bates' Guide to Physical Examination and History Taking, 9th ed. (Ch. 6, Tables of Abnormalities). Philadelphia, Lippincott Williams & Wilkins, 2007.

Chest Pain

Rakel RE. Conn's Current Therapy, 53rd ed. Philadelphia, WB Saunders, 2001.

Confusion

Bostwick JM. The many faces of confusion: timing and collateral history often hold the key to diagnosis. Postgraduate Medicine. 2000;108(6):60–72.

Marcantonio E. Section 5: Delirium and Dementia. Ch. 39: Disorders with unusual presentations in the elderly. In: The Merck Manual of Geriatrics, 1995–2001. Whitehouse Station, NJ, Merck and Company, Inc., USA, 2000.

Rajagopalan S, Yoshikawa T. Section 12: Kidney and Urinary Tract Disorders. Ch. 100: Urinary tract infections. In: The Merck Manual of Geriatrics, 1995–2001. Whitehouse Station, NJ, Merck and Company, Inc., USA, 2000.

Zawada E. Section 8: Metabolic and Endocrine Disorders. Ch. 57: Disorders of water and electrolyte balance; dehydration and volume depletion. In: The Merck Manual of Geriatrics, 1995–2001. Whitehouse Station, NJ, Merck and Company, Inc., USA, 2000.

Constipation

Goroll AH. Primary Care Medicine, 4th ed. Philadelphia, Lippincott Williams & Wilkins, 2000.

Acute Cough, Young Adult

MD Consult. First Consult. Available at: http://www.firstconsult.com/?type=med&id=01016540. Accessed April 7, 2005.

MD Consult. First Consult. Available at: http://www.firstconsult.com/?type=med&id=01014271. Accessed April 15, 2005.

Acute Cough, Older Adult

MD Consult. First Consult. Available at: http://www.firstconsult.com/?type=med&id=01014666. Accessed February 9, 2005.

Cough, Chronic

Drazen JM. Ch. 74: Asthma. In: Goldman L. Cecil Textbook of Medicine, 21st ed. Philadelphia, WB Saunders, 2000:393.

Rodante JR. Ch. 75: Chronic bronchitis and emphysema. In: Goldman L. Cecil Textbook of Medicine, 21st ed. Philadelphia, WB Saunders, 2000:394.

Dizziness

Hain TC, Micco A, Goetz CG. Meniere's disease. Ch. 12. Cranial Nerve VIII: vestibulocochlear system. In: Goetz CG. Textbook of Clinical Neurology. Philadelphia, WB Saunders, 1999.
Marill K. Vestibular neuronitis. eMedicine Journal. 2001;2(2).
Pruitt AA. Ch. 166: Evaluation of dizziness. In: Goroll AH. Primary Care Medicine, 4th ed. Philadelphia, Lippincott Williams & Wilkins, 2000.
Rakel RE. Conn's Current Therapy, 53rd ed. Philadelphia, WB Saunders, 2001.
Tusa RJ. Vertigo. Neurologic Clinics. 2001:19(1):23–55.
Yung WKA, Janus T. Ch 46: Neuroectodermal tumors: primary neurological tumors. In: Goetz CG. Textbook of Clinical Neurology. Philadelphia, WB Saunders, 1999:946.

Ear Pain

DeShazo R. Ch. 274. Allergic rhinitis. In: Goldman L. Cecil Textbook of Medicine, 21st ed. Philadelphia, WB Saunders, 2000:1446.
Klein JO. Ch. 50: Otitis externa, otitis media, mastoiditis. In: Mandell GL. Principles and Practice of Infectious Diseases, 5th ed. New York, Churchill Livingstone, 2000:670–674.
Schwartz RH. Otitis media. Rakel RE: In: Conn's Current Therapy, 53rd ed. Philadelphia, WB Saunders, 2001:213,214.
Slavin RG. Ch. 72: Nasal polyps and sinusitis. In: Middleton, Jr. Allergy: Principles and Practice, 5th ed. St. Louis, Mosby–Year Book, 1998:1027.

Fever

MD Consult. First Consult. Available at: http://www.firstconsult.com?type=med&id=01014561. Accessed March 23, 2005.
Leventhal WD, Hueston WJ, Virella G. Upper respiratory tract infections. In: Rakel RE. Textbook of Family Practice, 6th ed. Philadelphia, WB Saunders, 2001:350.
Mickelson SA, Benninger MS. Evaluation of Common Disorders. In Chapter 179: The nose and paranasal sinuses. In: Noble J. Textbook of Primary Care Medicine, 3rd ed. St. Louis, Mosby, Inc., 2001:1749.

Knee Pain

MD Consult. First Consult. Available at: http://www.firstconsult.com/?type=ddx&id=01220306. Accessed April 7, 2005.
Solomon DH, Simel DL, Bates DW, Katz JN, Schaffer JL. Does this patient have a torn meniscus or ligament of the knee? Value of the physical examination. JAMA. October 3, 2001;286(13):1610–20.

Leg Pain

Carman T, Fernandez BB Jr. A primary care approach to the patient with claudication. American Family Physician. 2000;61(4):1027–1032.
Creager MA, Libby P. Ch. 41: Peripheral arterial diseases. In: Braunwald E. Heart Disease: A Textbook of Cardiovascular Medicine, 6th ed. Philadelphia, WB Saunders, 2001:1462.

Loss of Vision

Frohman E. Vision and MS: What I need to know. Presented September 18, 2003, National Multiple Sclerosis Society. MS Learn Online. Available at: http://www.nationalmssociety.org/eduprog-specific.asp#vision.
Lam BL. Optic Neuritis and MS. Multiple Sclerosis Foundation. 2000–2003.
Wray SH. Optic Neuritis. Derzeitiger Forschungsstand zur Diagnose und Behandlung der Neuritis nervi optici, sowohl idiopathisch wie auch im Kontext der Multiplen Sklerose. Accessed April 28, 2005.

Low Back Pain

Biewen PC. A structured approach to low back pain: thorough evaluation is the key to effective treatment. Postgraduate Medicine. 1999;106(6):102–114.

Drezner JA, Herring SA. Managing low-back pain: steps to optimize function and hasten return to activity. The Physician and Sports Medicine. 2001;29(8).

Humphreys SC, Eck JC. Clinical evaluation and treatment options for herniated lumbar disc. American Family Physician. 1999;59(3):575–587.

Liu NYN, Caroso JJ. Ch.134: Periarticular rheumatic disorders. In: Noble J. Textbook of Primary Care Medicine, 3rd ed. St. Louis, Mosby, 2001:1251–1252.

Swenson R. Lower back pain: Differential diagnosis: a reasonable clinical approach. Neurologic Clinics. 1999;17(1):43–63.

Melanoma

Bickley LS. Bates' Guide to Physical Examination and History Taking, 9th ed. (Ch. 6, Tables of Abnormalities). Philadelphia, Lippincott Williams & Wilkins, 2007.

Memory Loss

MD Consult. First Consult. Available at: http://www.firstconsult.com/?type=ddx&id =01220357. Accessed April 24, 2005.

Brigham and Women's Hospital. Depression: a guide to diagnosis and treatment. Boston, Author, 2001. Available at: http://www.guideline.gov/summary/summary.aspx?ss=15&doc_id=3432& nbr=2658. Accessed May 8, 2005.

U.S. Department of Health and Human Services. Chapter 5: Older adults and mental health. Mental health: a report of the surgeon general. Rockville, MD, Author. Available at: http://www. surgeongeneral.gov/library/mentalhealth/chapter5/sec2.html#assessment. Accessed May 08, 2005.

Torpy JM, Writer; Cassio ML, Illustrator; Glass RM, Editor. JAMA Patient Page: Dementia. JAMA. September 22/29, 2004;292:1514.

Neck Pain

Campara B. Ch. 47: Soft tissue spine injuries and back pain. In: Marx JA. Rosen's Emergency Medicine: Concepts and Clinical Practice, 5th ed. St. Louis, Mosby–Year Book, 1998:601–611.

Palpitations

Englestein ED. Ch. 64: Ventricular arrhythmias in mitral valve prolapse. In: Zipes DP. Cardiac Electrophysiology, 3rd ed. Philadelphia, WB Saunders, 2000:563–568.

Hlatky MA. Ch 10: Approach to the patient with palpitations. In: Goldman L. and Brunwald E. Primary Cardiology. Philadelphia, WB Saunders, 1988:122–128.

Rash

The McGraw-Hill Companies. Systemic Lupus Erythematosus. How to manage, when to refer. Postgraduate Medicine. 2003;114(5). Available at: www.postgradmed.com. Accessed April 26, 2005.

Moses S. Malar Rash. Available at: http://www.fpnotebook.com/DER250.htm. Accessed April 25, 2005.

Eng MT, Cohen AS, Fries JF, et al. The 1982 Revised Criteria for the Classification of Systemic Lupus Erythematosus. The Arthritis Foundation: Arthritis and Rheumatism. 1982;25(11):1271–1277.

Rectal Bleeding

Fathi DJ. Office management of common anorectal problems. Common anorectal symptomatology. Primary Care: Clinics in Office Practice 1999;26(1):1–13.

Red Eye

Holmes HN. Professional Guide to Signs and Symptoms, 2nd ed. Springhouse, PA, Springhouse Corporation; 1997.

Shortness of Breath

MD Consult. First Consult. Available at: http://www.firstconsult.com/?type=med&id=01014666. Accessed February 9, 2005.

MD Consult. First Consult. Available at: http://www.firstconsult.com/?type=med&id=01016540. Accessed April 7, 2005.

MD Consult. First Consult. Available at: http://www.firstconsult.com/?type=med&id=01014271. Accessed April 15, 2005.

Shoulder Pain

Bickley LS. Bates' Guide to Physical Examination and History Taking, 9th ed. (Ch. 15, The Musculoskeletal System. Tables of Common Abnormalities: Tables 15-2 and 15-4) Philadelphia, Lippincott Williams & Wilkins, 2007.

MD Consult. First Consult. Available at: http://www.firstconsult.com/?type=ddx&id=01220318. Accessed April 7, 2005.

Sore Throat

Centers for Disease Control and Prevention. Careful antibiotic use: to avoid antibiotic resistance, treat only proven group A strep. Author.

Dowell SF, Schwartz B. Appropriate use of antibiotics for URIs in children: Part II. Cough, pharyngitis, and the common cold. American Family Physician. 1998;58(6):1113–1123.

Godshall SE, Kirchner JT. Infectious mononucleosis: complexities of a common syndrome. Postgraduate Medicine. 2000;107(7):175–186.

Ebell MH, Smith MA, Barry HC, Ives K, Carey M. The Rational Clinical Examination. Does this patient have strep throat? JAMA. 2000;284(22):2912–2918.

Hayes CS, Williamson H Jr. Management of group A beta hemolytic streptococcal pharyngitis. American Family Physician. 2001;63(8):1557–1565.

Stomach Pain

Agrawal S, Jonnalagadda S. Gallstones: From gallbladder to gut: management options for diverse complications. Postgraduate Medicine. 2000;108(3):143–153.

Bazaldua OV, Schneider FD. Table 1: In Differential diagnosis of dyspepsia. Evaluation and management of dyspepsia. American Family Physician. 1999;60(6).

Munoz A, Katerndahl DA. Diagnosis and management of acute pancreatitis. American Family Physician. 2000;62(1):164–174.

Unexplained Weight Loss

American Psychiatric Association. Diagnostic and Statistical Manual of Mental Disorders, 4th ed. Washington DC, Author, 1994.

Haddad G. Is it hyperthyroidism? You can't always tell from the clinical picture. Postgraduate Medicine. 1998;104(7).

Kaufman D, Longo DL. Hodgkin's disease: clinical manifestations. In: Abeloff MD. Clinical Oncology, 2nd ed. New York, Churchill Livingstone, 2000:2625–2627.

Urethral Discharge

Centers for Disease Control and Prevention. Management of male patients who have urethritis. Update on Sexually Transmitted Diseases. Author, 1998.

Roberts RG, Hartlaub PP. Evaluation of dysuria in men. American Family Physician. 1999;60(3):865–872.

Urinary Incontinence

MD Consult. First Consult. Available at: http://www.firsconsult.com/?type=ddx&id=01220337. Accessed April 24, 2005.

National Kidney and Urologic Diseases Information Clearinghouse. Urinary incontinence in women. Available at: http://kidney.niddk.nih.gov/kudiseases/pubs/uiwomen/index.htm Accessed May 8, 2005.

Vaginal Discharge

Bickley LS. Bates' Guide to Physical Examination and History Taking, 9th ed. (Ch. 11, Tables of Abnormalities). Lippincott Williams & Wilkins, 2007.

Wheezing

MD Consult. First Consult. Available at: http://www.firstconsult.com/?type=med&id=01014268. Accessed September 27, 2004.

Answers and Explanations

NOTE: Although additional portions of the physical examination may have been presented in the "actual findings" portion of the case studies, the parts of the physical examination listed in these answers are only those that are the most relevant to the patient's chief complaint and history of present

Chapter 1: Beginning the Physical Examination: General Survey and Vital Signs

CASE STUDIES

CASE STUDY: FEVER, ADULT

WHAT PARTS OF THE EXAM WOULD YOU LIKE TO PERFORM?

> General Survey
>
> Vital Signs
>
> Skin
>
> Head and Neck
>
> Thorax and Lungs
>
> Cardiovascular (limited)
>
> Abdomen (limited)

BASED ON THIS INFORMATION, WHAT IS YOUR DIFFERENTIAL DIAGNOSIS?

1. Meningitis
   Symptoms of meningitis include a sudden onset of severe, febrile systemic illness with confusion, obtundation, and neck stiffness, especially if the patient was previously healthy. Our patient presented to the office and was able to tell a coherent story, so there is no evidence of confusion or obtundation. Our patient complains of neck soreness, but on physical examination, there is no neck stiffness. In addition, she has no rash, which would be another symptom/sign in favor of meningitis.

2. Viral upper respiratory infection (URI)
   URIs are characterized by rhinorrhea, nasal congestion, sneezing, sore throat, and cough. The incubation period varies between 48 and 72 hours. In some cases, a low-grade fever is present, but temperature elevation in adults is rare. Episodes of colds are self-limited, with a median duration of 1 week. Most patients improve by the 10th day, but lingering symptoms may last up to 2 weeks.

3. Sinusitis (most likely diagnosis)
   Sinusitis typically presents with unilateral or bilateral nasal obstruction, purulent rhinorrhea, facial pain, and pressure overlying the paranasal sinuses. The pain is exacerbated with bending over or straining, and the maxillary teeth may be tender. Secretions may be clear (viral infection) or purulent (bacterial infection). Physical examination findings include tenderness to palpation over the paranasal sinuses, congestion of the turbinates, and purulent drainage in the nose, nasopharynx, or posterior oral pharynx. Transillumination of the sinuses may be performed but usually shows decreased light transmission of the involved sinus. In this case, the patient has persistent fever, so she may be partially dehydrated, which would cause the fever to linger.

CASE STUDY: UNEXPLAINED WEIGHT LOSS

WHAT PARTS OF THE EXAM WOULD YOU LIKE TO PERFORM?

> General Survey
>
> Vital Signs

Head and Neck

Cardiovascular

Musculoskeletal

Neurologic (including mental status)

BASED ON THIS INFORMATION, WHAT IS YOUR DIFFERENTIAL DIAGNOSIS?

1. Hodgkin's lymphoma

   This diagnosis, while possible, is less likely than some of the other possible etiologies. The patient has lost weight and has fever, night sweats, and low energy. She has not, however, noticed any swollen lymph nodes nor are any found on physical exam. Further testing would have to be done if this was a suspected diagnosis.

2. Hyperthyroidism

   Hyperthyroidism is the overproduction of thyroid hormone. There is no one single clinical indicator of hyperthyroidism. A constellation of several symptoms occurs that should increase your level of suspicion and lead you to further diagnostic testing. These include weight loss with preserved appetite, heat intolerance, nervousness, anxiety, insomnia, proximal muscle weakness, fatigue, tremor, heart palpitations, increased frequency of bowel movements, and decreased menstrual flow. Depression is less likely. Other general signs include hyperactivity, tachycardia or atrial fibrillation, systolic hypertension, lid lag, eyelid retraction, and hyper-reflexia. Although our patient has some of the symptoms of hyperthyroidism (e.g., weight loss despite a normal appetite, palpitations), she has none of the physical signs. In this situation, further testing would be required to make this diagnosis.

3. Depression (most likely diagnosis)

   Patients with severe depression may have significant weight loss. The specific diagnosis is made by asking about a constellation of symptoms: depressed mood or loss of interest or pleasure (anhedonia), along with significant weight loss when not dieting, or weight gain; insomnia or hypersomnia nearly every day; slower physical movements; fatigue or loss of energy; feelings of worthlessness or excessive or inappropriate guilt; a diminished ability to think or concentrate, or indecisiveness nearly every day; recurrent thoughts of death; and recurrent suicidal ideation with or without a specific plan. At least five of these symptoms must be present to make a diagnosis of depression.

MULTIPLE CHOICE

1. (D) Abdominal girth
2. (A) Sitting up
3. (A) Sitting up and leaning forward with arms braced
4. (B) He drank a cup of hot coffee just prior to having his temperature taken.
5. (D) Umbilicus

MATCHING

1. (E) Truncal fat: Cushing's syndrome
2. (A) Long limbs in proportion to the trunk: Marfan's syndrome
3. (B) Generalized fat: Obesity
4. (F) Very short stature: Turner's syndrome
5. (C) Exaggerated stare: Hyperthyroidism
6. (D) Masked facies: Parkinsonism

Chapter 2: The Skin, Hair, and Nails

CASE STUDIES

CASE STUDY: RASH

WHAT PARTS OF THE EXAM WOULD YOU LIKE TO PERFORM?

General Survey

Vital Signs

Skin

Head and Neck (limited)

Musculoskeletal

BASED ON THIS INFORMATION, WHAT IS YOUR DIFFERENTIAL DIAGNOSIS?

1. Lyme disease

   The patient has traveled to a location where she may be exposed to ticks and has fever and arthralgias, and the rash started in the appropriate time frame after possible exposure. The rash of Lyme disease, however, starts at the tick bite site and spreads centrifugally over days and weeks, and the lesions are not pruritic. Our patient's rash is not in the typical location.

2. Discoid lupus

   Discoid lupus typically has no systemic or constitutional symptoms, and our patient has fever and weight loss along with arthralgias. The rash is the same as that seen in systemic lupus erythematosus (SLE); however, the lesions are deeper into the dermis than the rash of SLE, so a biopsy would have to be performed to make the definitive diagnosis.

3. Systemic lupus erythematosus (most likely diagnosis)

   To definitively diagnose lupus, the patient must meet 4 out of 11 criteria as determined by the American College of Rheumatology. These criteria include physical examination findings, serological tests, and certain medical conditions. Our patient is in the appropriate age group for disease onset. In her history, she has constitutional symptoms such as fever and weight loss, as well as systemic symptoms such as arthralgias and increased sensitivity to the sun. On physical examination, she has a malar rash and oral ulcers.

Addendum: SLE Criteria (Need 4/11 to make the diagnosis):

- Malar rash
- Discoid rash
- Photosensitivity
- Oral ulcers
- Arthritis
- Two or more peripheral joints; tenderness, swelling or effusions; non-erosive
- Serositis
- Pleuritis/Pericarditis
- Renal disorder
- Proteinuria, cellular casts
- Neurologic disorder
- Seizures or psychosis
- Hematologic disorder
- Hemolytic anemia with reticulocytosis; leucopenia, lymphopenia, thrombocytopenia
- Immunologic disorder
- Positive LE cell preparation or anti-DNA ab, or Anti-Sm, or false-positive serologic test for syphilis
- ANA test

CASE STUDY: CHANGE IN MOLE

WHAT PARTS OF THE PHYSICAL EXAM WOULD YOU LIKE TO PERFORM?

   Vital Signs

   Skin

BASED ON THIS INFORMATION, WHAT IS YOUR DIFFERENTIAL DIAGNOSIS?

1. Squamous cell carcinoma

   This type of malignant skin cancer usually grows quickly and may develop in conjunction with an actinic keratosis. Squamous cell carcinoma typically appears on the sun-exposed skin of fair-skinned adults older than 60 years; the face or the backs of the hands are most often affected. Although Mr. C. is older than 60 years and the lesion is on his face, squamous cell carcinoma is firm and red and Mr. C.'s lesion is black; therefore, this is not the most likely of the differential diagnoses.

2. Basal cell carcinoma

   This type of malignant skin cancer grows slowly and seldom metastasizes. It is most common in fair-skinned adults older than 40 years, and it usually appears on the face. Initially, there is a translucent nodule that spreads, leaving a depressed center and a firm elevated border. Telangiectatic vessels are often visible.

3. Melanoma (most likely diagnosis)
   This is the most likely diagnosis for our patient. Melanoma is a highly malignant tumor that is most common in fair-skinned people. A possible warning sign is noticeable growth or color change in a benign nevus (mole). Additional suggestive signs are asymmetry, an irregular border, a diameter of more than 6 mm, and an elevated, irregular surface (the ABCDEs). Confirmation would require biopsy of the lesion.

MULTIPLE CHOICE

1. (A) Central cyanosis
2. (C) Jaundice
3. (A) Cool
4. (D) Diameter smaller than 6 mm
5. (A) Basal cell carcinoma

MATCHING

1. (B) Macule: Small spot
2. (D) Papule: Palpable elevated mass up to 0.5 cm in diameter; solid
3. (A) Vesicle: Circumscribed superficial elevation up to 0.5 cm in diameter; filled with serous fluid
4. (C) Basal cell carcinoma: Initially translucent nodule; spreads; leaves a depressed center with a firm elevated border
5. (F) Squamous cell carcinoma: May develop in conjunction with an actinic keratosis; firm, red
6. (E) Spider angioma: Fiery red; central body surrounded by erythema and radiating legs

Chapter 3: The Head and Neck

CASE STUDIES

CASE STUDY: RED AND BURNING EYES

WHAT PARTS OF THE EXAM WOULD YOU LIKE TO PERFORM?

General Survey
Vital Signs
Head and Neck
Skin

BASED ON THIS INFORMATION, WHAT IS YOUR DIFFERENTIAL DIAGNOSIS?

1. Conjunctivitis
   This illness is typically preceded by or accompanies an upper respiratory infection; the pain is usually described as mild discomfort, and visual acuity is unaffected. The pupillary response is normal and the cornea is clear. Watery, mucoid, or mucopurulent ocular discharge is usually present.
2. Corneal injury
   Although the patient works as a machinist and may have had a work-related exposure to sparks (which can cause flash burns) or metal fragments, this is not the most likely diagnosis. The pain associated with a corneal injury is usually described as moderate to severe and is superficial. The pupil is not affected and usually there is no cloudiness to the cornea. There may be a watery or purulent ocular discharge.
3. Glaucoma (most likely diagnosis)
   Patients describe the pain of acute angle-closure glaucoma as severe, aching, and deep. Visual acuity is decreased, and the affected pupil is typically dilated and fixed. The cornea may be steamy or cloudy. Ocular discharge is absent. Acute angle-closure glaucoma is a medical emergency, and the patient must be referred immediately to an ophthalmologist.

CASE STUDY: EAR PAIN

WHAT PARTS OF THE EXAM WOULD YOU LIKE TO PERFORM?

General Survey
Vital Signs

Skin

Head and Neck

Thorax and Lungs

Cardiovascular (limited)

BASED ON THIS INFORMATION, WHAT IS YOUR DIFFERENTIAL DIAGNOSIS?

1. Sinusitis

   This is a condition that may be caused by a viral or bacterial infection. Typical features of the history are malaise or fatigue, fever, nasal discharge that is purulent, and cough. On physical examination, there may be retraction of the tympanic membrane secondary to increased rhinorrhea; the sinuses may be tender to palpation. The nasal mucosa may be erythematous and swollen. Because Johnny has no nasal congestion, change in color of the nasal mucosa, sinus tenderness, or retraction of the tympanic membrane, this is not the most likely diagnosis.

2. Allergic rhinitis

   Typically, there is no fever in allergic rhinitis. The nasal discharge is clear, and the patient may complain of itchy eyes, with a clear discharge. On physical examination, the tympanic membranes are shiny or may be slightly retracted; the nasal mucosa is pale and boggy.

3. Otitis media (most likely diagnosis)

   The classic sign of otitis media is an erythematous, bulging tympanic membrane. There may be a meniscus level, indicating fluid behind the tympanic membrane. Otitis media may or may not be accompanied by fever; if the child is older than 5 years, then fever may not be present. Most cases of otitis media are caused by viruses; if bacteria are involved, then the most common bacterial agents are Streptococcus pneumoniae, Haemophilus influenzae, and Moraxella catarrhalis.

CASE STUDY: SORE THROAT

WHAT PARTS OF THE EXAM WOULD YOU LIKE TO PERFORM?

General Survey

Vital Signs

Skin

Head and Neck

Thorax and Lungs

Cardiovascular (limited)

Abdomen

BASED ON THIS INFORMATION, WHAT IS YOUR DIFFERENTIAL DIAGNOSIS?

1. Mononucleosis

   Fever, pharyngitis, and lymphadenopathy are the classic triad of symptoms and signs for mononucleosis, which is most common in the adolescent and young adult age groups. Other symptoms of infectious mononucleosis are fatigue, malaise, and sore throat. Typical physical examination findings are diffuse exudates on the tonsil and enlargement of the posterior cervical lymph nodes (typically more so than in a bacterial infection). Palatal petechiae and enlargement of the spleen may also be present. Mononucleosis is not, however, the most likely diagnosis for our patient, who is only 7 years old. Additionally, her lymphadenopathy is anterior, not posterior, and she lacks palatal petechiae.

2. Viral pharyngitis

   According to the Centers for Disease Control and Prevention (CDC), clinical findings alone do not adequately distinguish streptococcal pharyngitis from non-streptococcal pharyngitis. There are symptom scores that help to increase the suspicion for viral pharyngitis when compared to strep. If the patient has prominent rhinorrhea, cough, hoarseness, conjunctivitis, or diarrhea, then a viral etiology is more likely. Our patient has a clear nasal discharge and a nonproductive cough; this increases the likelihood of a viral pharyngitis. If we were concerned about the presence of a streptococcal infection in our patient, then we would proceed with further testing (i.e., rapid strep test or throat culture).

3. Streptococcal pharyngitis (most likely diagnosis)

   According to the CDC, clinical findings alone do not adequately distinguish streptococcal pharyngitis from nonstreptococcal pharyngitis. There are symptom scores that have been developed that help to increase or decrease the suspicion for strep. The Centor Clinical

Prediction rule for diagnosis of strep has shown that if the patient has three out of the following four symptoms, then he or she has a higher likelihood of having strep: history of fever, anterior cervical adenopathy, tonsillar exudate, and absence of cough. Our patient has very similar findings to those associated with streptococcal pharyngitis; however, she has clear rhinorrhea and a nonproductive cough, which would go against the diagnosis of streptococcal pharyngitis. Further testing would have to be performed to confirm the presence of streptococcus.

MULTIPLE CHOICE

1. (A) Fine texture
2. (C) Dry, flaking areas on the scalp
3. (C) Coarsening of the facial features
4. (B) Protrusion
5. (D) Bitemporal hemianopsia
6. (A) Absence of the red reflex
7. (B) Arteriovenous (AV) nicking
8. (B) Anisocoria
9. (A) Horner's syndrome
10. (A) Umbo
11. (A) Erythematous, bulging tympanic membrane
12. (D) Otitis externa
13. (A) Weber's test
14. (B) Rinne's test
15. (B) Pale to bluish boggy mucosa
16. (B) White plaques
17. (A) Exudates on the tonsils
18. (A) Thyroiditis
19. (B) Place your index fingers above the cricoid cartilage

MATCHING
EYES

1. (C) Pupillary reaction to light: CN II (optic) and CN III (oculomotor)
2. (E) Anisocoria: Pupillary inequality of less than 0.5 mm
3. (A) Extraocular motion: CN III (oculomotor), CN IV (trochlear), and CN VI (abducens)
4. (B) Blind spot: 15 degrees temporal to the line of gaze
5. (D) Normal visual acuity: 20/20

EARS

6. (B) Weber's test: Lateralization of sound with tuning fork
7. (A) Rinne's test: Normally air conduction is two times longer than bone conduction
8. (D) Enables optimal examination of adult's tympanic membrane: External ear pulled downward, backward, and slightly away from the head
9. (C) Enables optimal examination of infant's tympanic membrane: External ear pulled downward, outward, and backward

NOSE

10. (A,C) Turbinates visible on inspection: Middle turbinate, inferior turbinate
11. (D,E) Sinuses that are palpable: Maxillary sinus, frontal sinus

MOUTH AND PHARYNX

12. (A) Normal number of adult teeth: 32
13. (E) Raises soft palate: CN X (vagus)
14. (D) Enables tongue protrusion: CN XII (hypoglossal)

NECK

15. (B) Anterior triangle boundaries: Mandible, sternomastoid muscle, midline of neck
16. (A) Posterior triangle boundaries: Sternomastoid muscle, trapezius muscle, clavicle

17. (F) Normal position of the trachea: Midline
18. (E) Palpation of the thyroid gland: Below the cricoid cartilage
19. (C) Enlarged thyroid gland: Presence of a bruit

Chapter 4: The Thorax and Lungs

CASE STUDIES

CASE STUDY: ACUTE COUGH, YOUNG ADULT

WHAT PARTS OF THE EXAM WOULD YOU LIKE TO PERFORM?

General Survey
Vital Signs
Head and Neck
Thorax and Lungs
Cardiovascular (limited)

BASED ON THIS INFORMATION, WHAT IS YOUR DIFFERENTIAL DIAGNOSIS?

1. Pneumothorax
   Pneumothorax is characterized by shortness of breath and pleuritic pain. On physical examination, there is tracheal deviation, diminished expansion on the affected side, and diminished breath sounds and hyperresonance with percussion. Our patient does not have pleuritic pain, and both sides are affected in her disease condition, not just one side.
2. COPD
   COPD is characterized by a chronic cough with any pattern of chronic sputum production. The chronic cough must be present for at least 2 years before the diagnosis can be made. Our patient has had the cough for only 5 days. The patient experiences dyspnea and breathlessness that is progressive, persistent, worse with exercise, and worse during respiratory infections. Our patient does not have a progressive disease process. Upon physical examination, wheezing (nonspecific and variable), delayed expiratory phase, decreased breath sounds, and signs of lung hyperinflation are present. Our patient has wheezing, with delayed expiratory phase and decreased breath sounds, but her thorax is symmetric with a normal AP diameter, which is not consistent with COPD.
3. Asthma (most likely diagnosis)
   Asthma is reversible airway inflammation and broncho-constriction characterized by episodic wheezing, dyspnea, cough (chronic, dry, and often nocturnal), poor exercise tolerance, and a feeling of tightness in the chest. This results from airway hypersensitivity in response to stimuli, such as smoke, exercise, or cold air. Our patient has a childhood history of asthma. She is 29 years old, and asthma is more common than COPD in a younger adult. She also appears to have the trigger of a respiratory infection. Upon physical examination, prolonged expiration and diffuse high-pitched wheezes are noted, which is consistent with our patient's presentation.

CASE STUDY: ACUTE COUGH, OLDER ADULT

WHAT PARTS OF THE EXAM WOULD YOU LIKE TO PERFORM?

General Survey
Vital Signs
Skin
Head and Neck
Thorax and Lungs

BASED ON THIS INFORMATION, WHAT IS YOUR DIFFERENTIAL DIAGNOSIS?

1. Lung cancer
   Common symptoms of lung cancer include the following: cough (usually dry and persistent), dyspnea (with or without wheezing), hemoptysis, weight loss, anorexia, fatigue, chest pains, muscle weakness or pain, and confusion and memory loss. Common signs include: lobar consolidation, localized wheezing, pleural effusion, tracheal shift or tug, cachexia, lymphadenopathy, hepatomegaly, ascites, and clubbing. Our patient lacks hemoptysis, chest pains, muscle

weakness or pain, confusion or memory loss. He does not have localized wheezing, tracheal shift or tug, cachexia, lymphadenopathy, hepatomegaly, ascites, or clubbing. He is therefore less likely to have lung cancer, although his history of chewing tobacco may make you want to investigate this possibility and consider a chest X-ray if this infection does not resolve.

2. Bronchitis
   The main signs of acute bronchitis are productive cough worse with exercise or lying down, and wheezing. It is often with an associated upper respiratory tract infection. The patient may have a normal temperature or a low-grade fever. The sputum is usually clear or white. Patients generally do have the flushed toxic appearance of a systemic infection.

3. Lobar pneumonia (most likely)
   Our patient has a productive cough with purulent sputum as well as subjective shortness of breath and chest pain. These symptoms are consistent with a respiratory infection, which is more serious than bronchitis. Our patient has fever during his examination, although he denied any subjective sense of fever or chills. He is also tachypneic and tachycardic. He has diminished breath sounds to auscultation along with dullness to percussion over the affected lobe. In addition to this, the area is positive for egophony, which is highly suggestive of a consolidation.

CASE STUDY: SHORTNESS OF BREATH

WHAT PARTS OF THE EXAM WOULD YOU LIKE TO PERFORM?

General Survey

Vital Signs

Head and Neck

Thorax and Lungs

Cardiovascular

BASED ON THIS INFORMATION, WHAT IS YOUR DIFFERENTIAL DIAGNOSIS?

1. Lung cancer
   Common symptoms of lung cancer include the following: cough (usually dry and persistent), dyspnea (with or without wheezing), hemoptysis, weight loss, anorexia, fatigue, chest pains, muscle weakness or pain, and confusion and memory loss. Common signs include lobar consolidation, localized wheezing, pleural effusion, tracheal shift or tug, cachexia, lymphadenopathy, hepatomegaly, ascites, and clubbing. Our patient lacks hemoptysis, chest pains, muscle weakness or pain, and confusion or memory loss. He does not have a lobar consolidation by percussion of his lung fields; he does not have localized wheezing, tracheal shift or tug, cachexia, lymphadenopathy, hepatomegaly, ascites, or clubbing. He is therefore less likely to have lung cancer, although his history of smoking and his weight loss make further testing indicated.

2. Asthma
   Asthma is characterized by *episodic* wheezing, dyspnea, cough (chronic, dry, and often nocturnal), poor exercise tolerance, and a feeling of tightness in the chest. This results from airway hypersensitivity in response to stimuli, such as smoke, exercise, or cold air. Upon physical examination, prolonged expiration and diffuse high-pitched wheezes are noted. Our patient has a productive cough that is not nocturnal, and he denies chest tightness; there are also no obvious triggers in his situation. Changes in the AP diameter of the thorax are much less likely in patients with asthma.

3. COPD (most likely diagnosis)
   COPD is characterized by a chronic cough with any pattern of chronic sputum production. The patient experiences dyspnea and breathlessness that is progressive, persistent, worse with exercise, and worse during respiratory infections. The patient may also experience some nonspecific and variable chest tightness. Upon physical examination, wheezing (nonspecific and variable), delayed expiratory phase, decreased breath sounds, and signs of lung hyperinflation are present. The patient may lose weight secondary to the increased metabolic demands of untreated COPD.

CASE STUDY: COUGH, CHRONIC

WHAT PARTS OF THE EXAM WOULD YOU LIKE TO PERFORM?

General Survey

Vital Signs

Skin
Head and Neck
Thorax and Lungs
Cardiovascular

BASED ON THIS INFORMATION, WHAT IS YOUR DIFFERENTIAL DIAGNOSIS?

1. Chronic obstructive pulmonary disease (COPD) exacerbation
   There are two forms of COPD: emphysema and chronic bronchitis. The patient does not give a history of productive cough for at least 3 weeks, which is the definition of chronic bronchitis. Additionally, he has a fever and his sputum production is not merely increased—it is also of a different color, suggesting an infectious process.
2. Asthma
   Asthma is a reversible airway disease. Patients usually exhibit signs of this illness before the age of 40. The signs are wheezing and, often, a chronic cough that may or may not be productive. The fact that our patient's cough is productive of green, blood-tinged sputum suggests that this is not an asthma exacerbation.
3. Acute bronchitis (most likely diagnosis)
   This patient has a fever with a cough productive of green, blood-tinged sputum, making infection the most likely answer. Infections will also cause hyperreactivity of the airways and result in wheezing. Pneumonia could be considered, but there are no areas of dullness over the lung fields, suggesting consolidation.

MULTIPLE CHOICE

1. (B) Increased
2. (A) Dull
3. (B) "AAY"
4. (B) Egophony
5. (A) Increased AP diameter
6. (B) Delayed expiratory phase
7. (B) Increased resonance (hyperresonance) on the affected side
8. (C) Absent breath sounds
9. (B) 5 to 6 cm
10. (C) 14 to 20 breaths per minute

MATCHING

1. (E) Location, anteriorly, of lower border of lung: Sixth rib, midclavicular line, and eighth rib, axillary line
2. (C) Location, posteriorly, of lower border of lung: T10 spinous process
3. (B) Trachea bifurcation: Sternal angle anteriorly and T4 spinous process posteriorly
4. (D) Fremitus: Palpable vibrations transmitted through the bronchopulmonary tree to the chest wall when the patient speaks
5. (A) Location of broncho-vesicular breath sounds: First and second interspaces anteriorly and between the scapulae

Chapter 5: The Cardiovascular System

CASE STUDIES

CASE STUDY: CHEST PAIN

WHAT PARTS OF THE EXAM WOULD YOU LIKE TO PERFORM?

General Survey
Vital Signs
Skin
Head and Neck
Thorax and Lungs
Cardiovascular
Peripheral Vascular/Extremities

BASED ON THIS INFORMATION, WHAT IS YOUR MOST LIKELY DIFFERENTIAL DIAGNOSIS?

1. Peptic ulcer

   The pain of peptic ulcer disease can be in the epigastric area of the upper abdomen or in the lower precordial region of the chest. On physical examination, there is usually mild tenderness in the epigastric region. However, ulcer pain is unlikely to arise from exertion or to be accompanied by sweating.

2. Aortic dissection

   The chest pain of aortic dissection is typically described as "tearing" in nature; it is located in the precordium but can radiate into the back or up the side of the neck. Upon physical examination, blood pressure in the arms may be unequal and there may be an inequality of pulses in the upper extremities when compared with the lower extremities. You may also hear the murmur of aortic regurgitation. In our patient's case, the chest pain is not "tearing" and the blood pressure is equal in both arms, so this is not the most likely diagnosis.

3. Acute myocardial infarction (most likely diagnosis)

   In acute myocardial infarction, the classic description of cardiac pain is that of chest pressure or tightness. Typically, the pain is substernal in the midprecordium, with radiation into the left neck, jaw, shoulder, or arm. This patient also has multiple risk factors for cardiovascular disease, including hypertension, smoking, and a family history of the early onset of cardiac disease (both his father and paternal grandfather died of acute myocardial infarction before the age of 50).

CASE STUDY: PALPITATIONS

WHAT PARTS OF THE EXAM WOULD YOU LIKE TO PERFORM?

General Survey

Vital Signs

Skin

Head and Neck

Thorax and Lungs

Cardiovascular

Peripheral Vascular/ Extremities

BASED ON THIS INFORMATION, WHAT IS YOUR DIFFERENTIAL DIAGNOSIS?

1. Heightened awareness of normal heartbeat

   This patient has a midsystolic click, so a cardiac finding is present. In general, when you perform your physical examination, you will be looking for evidence of underlying cardiac disease, regardless of the type of palpitation. Physical findings that confirm evidence of cardiac disease include rales, an elevated JVP, valvular murmurs, an S3, or peripheral edema.

2. Premature ventricular contractions

   The heart rate would be irregular, and you would not expect a midsystolic click. The patient usually does not experience worsening of palpitations with exercise; symptoms may worsen with caffeine intake. An electrocardiogram is needed for the diagnosis of any arrhythmias.

3. Mitral valve prolapse (most likely diagnosis)

   The classic sign of mitral valve prolapse (MVP) is a midsystolic click, best heard at or medial to the apex but also discernible at the lower left sternal border in some patients. The midsystolic click may or may not be followed by a late systolic murmur. The "classic" patient is a young woman. The symptoms of palpitations are often accompanied by anxiety.

MULTIPLE CHOICE

1. (A) An irregularly irregular rhythm
2. (C) 6 cm above the sternal angle
3. (B) A midsystolic click
4. (A) Perform a Valsalva maneuver
5. (B) PMI in the fifth interspace, anterior axillary line

MATCHING
HEART SOUNDS

1. (B) S1: Produced by closure of the mitral valve
2. (D) S2: Produced by closure of the aortic valve

3. (C) S3: Occurs after the mitral valve opens; rapid ventricular filling
4. (A) S4: Occurs during atrial contraction

MURMURS

5. (C) Grade VI murmur: May be heard when the stethoscope is entirely off the chest
6. (B) Grade I murmur: Very faint
7. (A) Grade IV murmur: Loud; may be associated with a thrill

VALVE DISORDERS

8. (D) Aortic stenosis: Midsystolic; crescendo–decrescendo murmur
9. (C) Mitral regurgitation: Pan-systolic; plateau murmur
10. (A) Mitral valve stenosis: Mid- to late systolic; opening snap
11. (B) Aortic regurgitation: Early diastolic; decrescendo murmur

LABELING

1. Second right interspace (aortic)
2. Second left interspace (pulmonic)
3. Apex (mitral)
4. Lower left sternal border (tricuspid)

Chapter 6: The Breasts and Axillae

CASE STUDY

CASE STUDY: LUMP

WHAT PARTS OF THE EXAM WOULD YOU LIKE TO PERFORM?
General Survey
Vital Signs
Skin
Breasts and Axillae

BASED ON THIS INFORMATION, WHAT IS YOUR DIFFERENTIAL DIAGNOSIS?
1. Fibroadenoma
A fibroadenoma is usually found in patients between the ages of 15 and 25 years but may be seen in patients as old as 55 years. Fibroadenomas are round, disclike, or lobular. They are usually firm in consistency, well delineated, and mobile. Tenderness is usually absent. Retraction of the skin does not occur. Fibroadenomas are less likely to change with menses.
2. Breast cancer
Breast cancer is rare in 30-year-old women. With breast cancer, there may be dimpling of the skin, but this patient has no changes in the skin over her breasts. The lump is usually irregular or stellate in shape and has a firm or hard consistency. The lump may not be well delineated from the surrounding tissues. The patient has no palpable adenopathy in the axillary, infraclavicular, or supraclavicular lymph nodes, which may occur if breast cancer is metastatic.
3. Cyst (most likely diagnosis)
Cysts typically appear in women between the ages of 30 and 50 years and regress after menopause. There may be one cyst or multiple cysts. Cysts are round, soft to firm in consistency, and usually elastic; they are well delineated and mobile. They are often tender to the touch, and there are no signs of retraction. Cysts may change in shape with the menstrual cycle. Although this is the most likely diagnosis for our patient, all breast lumps raise the concern of breast cancer and warrant careful evaluation and follow-up.

MULTIPLE CHOICE

1. (B) Cyst
2. (C) Fibrocystic breast disease

MATCHING

1. (D) Fibroadenoma: Fine, round, mobile, nontender
2. (A) Cyst: Soft to firm, round, mobile, often tender
3. (B) Fibrocystic changes: Nodular, ropelike
4. (C) Breast cancer: Irregular, stellate, firm, not clearly delineated from surrounding tissue

Chapter 7: The Abdomen

CASE STUDY

CASE STUDY: STOMACH PAIN

WHAT PARTS OF THE EXAM WOULD YOU LIKE TO PERFORM?

General Survey

Vital Signs

Skin

Thorax and Lungs

Cardiovascular

Abdomen

BASED ON THIS INFORMATION, WHAT IS YOUR DIFFERENTIAL DIAGNOSIS?

1. Peptic ulcer

   This condition is characterized by midepigastric pain and, at times, by right upper quadrant pain. The pain may radiate to the back and is variable in quality—patients may describe it as "gnawing," "burning," "boring," "aching," "pressure," or "hunger-like." The pain may be worse after eating or relieved by eating, depending on the location of the ulcer. The pain associated with peptic ulcer can be difficult to distinguish from that associated with chole-cystitis, and further testing may be required. Risk factors for peptic ulcers include the use of nonsteroidal anti-inflammatory drugs (NSAIDs) or aspirin, cigarette smoking, and a family history of ulcers. This is not the most likely diagnosis for our patient, however. She has intermittent spasms of pain rather than gnawing pain. Additionally, her symptoms are associated with eating fatty foods, whereas in peptic ulcer disease, eating food in general (not just fatty food) affects symptoms.

2. Pancreatitis

   This condition is characterized by epigastric or left upper quadrant pain that radiates to the back. The pain is usually described as severe, constant, dull, and boring. It is worse when the patient is supine and may lessen when the patient assumes a sitting or a fetal position. It is usually accompanied by nausea and vomiting. The pain is typically associated with a recent intake of alcohol or a heavy meal. On physical examination, there may be abdominal distension and epigastric and left upper quadrant tenderness, but no Murphy's sign. Other signs such as fever, tachycardia, and jaundice may be present. Also, this patient has intermittent rather than constant pain.

3. Biliary colic (most likely diagnosis)

   The pain associated with biliary colic is likely to occur after a meal, especially one high in fat. The pain is located in the epigastric region, or the right upper quadrant. It is often described as severe, steady, and aching, and it may last several hours; it may radiate to the right scapula. The pain increases in intensity over 15 minutes, reaches a plateau, and then may last up to 6 hours. Most episodes are accompanied by nausea and vomiting. There is often a family history of cholelithiasis. Biliary colic typically occurs in women who are obese and in their 40s. Upon physical examination, mild to moderate tenderness of the right upper quadrant may be present during inspiration (a positive Murphy's sign). Unlike cholecystitis, biliary colic is not usually associated with fever, and the pain lessens spontaneously.

MULTIPLE CHOICE

1. (A) Inspection, auscultation, percussion, palpation
2. (D) Voluntary guarding
3. (C) Rovsing's sign

4. (B) CVA tenderness
5. (C) Murphy's sign
6. (A) Liver edge is tender and 4 to 5 finger-breadths below the RCM

MATCHING

1. (B) Liver edge: Palpable 6 cm below the right costal margin in the midclavicular line during inspiration
2. (A) Spleen edge: Palpable deep to the left costal margin during inspiration
3. (F) Rovsing's sign: Pain in the right lower quadrant during palpation of the left lower quadrant
4. (D) Psoas sign: Examiner's hand is placed on the patient's right knee and the patient is asked to raise his or her right thigh against the examiner's hand
5. (C) Obturator sign: Pain elicited when the patient's right thigh is flexed at the hip with the knee bent, and the leg is internally rotated at the hip
6. (E) Cutaneous hyperesthesia: Pain elicited by gently picking up a fold of abdominal skin anteriorly

LABELING

1. Liver
2. Gallbladder
3. Duodenum
4. Spleen
5. Stomach
6. Pancreas
7. Costovertebral angle
8. Eleventh rib
9. Twelfth rib
10. Kidney
11. Aorta
12. Renal artery
13. Iliac artery
14. Femoral artery

Chapter 8: Male Genitalia and Hernias

CASE STUDY

CASE STUDY: URETHRAL DISCHARGE

WHAT PARTS OF THE PHYSICAL EXAM WOULD YOU LIKE TO PERFORM?

General Survey

Vital Signs

Skin

Abdomen

Male Genitalia

Anus, Rectum, and Prostate

BASED ON THIS INFORMATION, WHAT IS YOUR DIFFERENTIAL DIAGNOSIS?

1. Epididymitis
   Epididymitis is associated with pain on palpation of the posterolateral surface of the epididymis. Epididymitis is usually unilateral, and one of the presenting symptoms is "scrotal heaviness." Urethral discharge may or may not be present. Because this patient has no tenderness upon palpation of the testes or epididymis, epididymitis is a less likely diagnosis.
2. Prostatitis
   Prostatitis may be associated with rectal pain and tenderness upon palpation of the prostate. The prostate may feel "boggy." Physical examination may reveal enlargement of the prostate. Prostatitis may or may not be associated with sexual activity. Typically, there is no

purulent urethral discharge. Furthermore, this patient has no tenderness upon palpation of the prostate.
3. Urethritis, Chlamydia (most likely diagnosis)
Urethritis, or inflammation of the urethra, is caused by an infection and is characterized by the discharge of mucopurulent or purulent material and by burning during urination. Urethritis is the sexually transmitted disease (STD) that most frequently affects men in developed countries. Asymptomatic infections are common. According to the Centers for Disease Control and Prevention (CDC) (in Atlanta), the only bacterial pathogens of proven clinical importance in men who have urethritis are Neisseria gonorrhoeae and Chlamydia trachomatis. Chlamydia trachomatis is the most common cause, isolated in 23% to 55% of cases.

MULTIPLE CHOICE

1. (C) Hernia
2. (D) Genital herpes
3. (A) Hydrocele
4. (B) Testicular torsion

MATCHING

1. (D) Phimosis: Tight prepuce that cannot be retracted over the glans
2. (C) Paraphimosis: Tight prepuce; once retracted, cannot be returned
3. (E) Balanitis: Inflammation of the glans
4. (B) Hypospadias: Ventral displacement of the urethral meatus on the penis
5. (A) Cryptorchidism: Undescended testicle

Chapter 9: Female Genitalia

CASE STUDY

CASE STUDY: VAGINAL DISCHARGE

WHAT PARTS OF THE PHYSICAL EXAM WOULD YOU LIKE TO PERFORM?

General Survey
Vital Signs
Skin
Abdomen
Female Genitalia

BASED ON THIS INFORMATION, WHAT IS YOUR DIFFERENTIAL DIAGNOSIS?

1. Candida vaginitis
This is a yeast infection, and, although it is associated with a discharge, the discharge is typically white, curdlike, and without odor. It may be thin or thick in consistency. There is itching, vaginal soreness, pain on urination, and dyspareunia, due to inflammation of the skin. The vulva and vaginal mucosa are often red. To definitively diagnose a yeast infection, further confirmation is needed. A sample of the discharge added to a drop of potassium hydroxide (KOH) on a glass slide will reveal branching hyphae under the microscope.
2. Pelvic inflammatory disease
This disease typically has more symptoms than an isolated vaginal discharge. The patient may have fever and pelvic pain. On physical examination, there may be tender, bilateral adnexal masses or cervical motion tenderness. A yellow purulent discharge is common in the cervical os. Typical causative organisms are Neisseria gonorrhoeae and Chlamydia trachomatis. If ulcerating lesions are present, then herpes simplex should be considered. Diagnosis is based on Gram stain and culture.
3. Bacterial vaginosis (most likely diagnosis)
The organisms that cause this bacterial infection are not well identified. Bacterial vaginosis may be transmitted sexually but is not considered an STD. The discharge is gray, white, thin, homogeneous, and malodorous, and it coats the vaginal walls. The odor has been described as fishy or musty. The vulva and vaginal mucosa are normal in appearance. Further

confirmation is needed to make the diagnosis. A sample of the discharge added to a drop of normal saline on a glass slide will reveal clue cells (epithelial cells with stippled borders) under the microscope; a drop of potassium hydroxide (KOH) will elicit a fishy odor (positive "whiff" test).

MULTIPLE CHOICE

1. (C) Candida vaginitis
2. (B) Venereal warts
3. (A) Leiomyoma or fibroid
4. (D) Tubo-ovarian abscess

LABELING

1. Mons pubis
2. Prepuce
3. Clitoris
4. Urethral meatus
5. Opening of paraurethral (Skene's) gland
6. Vestibule
7. Introitus
8. Perineum
9. Labium majus
10. Labium minus
11. Hymen
12. Vagina
13. Opening of Bartholin's gland
14. Anus

Chapter 10: The Anus, Rectum, and Prostate

CASE STUDIES

CASE STUDY: CONSTIPATION

WHAT PARTS OF THE EXAM WOULD YOU LIKE TO PERFORM?

General Survey

Vital Signs

Skin

Thorax and Lungs

Cardiovascular

Anus, Rectum, and Prostate

BASED ON THIS INFORMATION, WHAT IS YOUR DIFFERENTIAL DIAGNOSIS?

1. Hypothyroidism
   Constipation is one symptom of hypothyroidism, but other systemic symptoms are usually present, such as fatigue, decreased ability to concentrate, depression, coarsening of hair, and increased weight. Upon physical examination, a rectal mass is not present, and the stool is usually not guaiac-positive, so this is not the most likely diagnosis for Mr. H.

2. Depression
   Elderly patients often experience depression with constitutional symptoms such as constipation, weight loss, and fatigue. They may report increased confusion, withdrawal from normal activities, and decreased appetite. Physical examination would be normal, except for a flat affect. Although Mr. H. has experienced constitutional symptoms such as weight loss and diminished appetite, and he no longer participates in activities that he used to enjoy (due to lack of energy), depression is not the most likely diagnosis given the physical examination findings.

3. Colon cancer (most likely diagnosis)
   Given the patient's age and history of changes in bowel habits, decreased appetite, and weight loss, and the palpable mass upon rectal examination with a guaiac-positive stool, colon cancer is the most likely diagnosis until proven otherwise by further testing.

CASE STUDY: RECTAL BLEEDING, OLDER ADULT

WHAT PARTS OF THE EXAM WOULD YOU LIKE TO PERFORM?

General Survey

Vital Signs

Skin

Cardiovascular

Abdomen

Anus, Rectum, and Prostate

BASED ON THIS INFORMATION, WHAT IS YOUR DIFFERENTIAL DIAGNOSIS?

1. Internal hemorrhoids
   Internal hemorrhoids are almost always associated with painless bleeding. Usually, bright red blood appears on the bowel movement in small amounts and is described as staining the toilet paper or coloring the toilet bowl. This patient passed dark red blood and has no history of constipation.
2. Colon cancer
   This is a less likely diagnosis; most colon cancer is asymptomatic until the cancer is large enough to present as a bowel obstruction (either partial or complete). There may be bleeding but not usually in a massive amount acutely. Because colon cancer is often asymptomatic, screening with flexible sigmoidoscopy or colonoscopy is recommended after age 50.
3. Diverticulosis (most likely diagnosis)
   Diverticular disease is more common with advancing age and is the most common cause of massive lower gastrointestinal bleeding in adults. The bleeding is generally painless. It is important to assess the patient for hemodynamic stability (i.e., stable pulse, blood pressure, respirations) and to consider hospital admission.

CASE STUDY: RECTAL BLEEDING, YOUNG ADULT

WHAT PARTS OF THE EXAM WOULD YOU LIKE TO PERFORM?

General Survey

Vital Signs

Abdomen

Anus, Rectum, and Prostate

BASED ON THIS INFORMATION, WHAT IS YOUR DIFFERENTIAL DIAGNOSIS?

1. Colon cancer
   This is a less likely diagnosis, given the lack of family history of colon cancer, the lack of constitutional symptoms, and the absence of guaiac-positive stools. Further testing would be needed to rule out this diagnosis if there is a stronger suspicion.
2. Anal fissure
   An anal fissure is a very painful ulceration of the anal canal, found most commonly in the midline posteriorly and less commonly in the midline anteriorly. There may be a swollen "sentinel" skin tag just below the fissure, and gentle separation of the anal margins may reveal its lower edge. The sphincter is spastic, and the examination is painful. This patient has no pain with defecation, no visible fissure on examination, and no rectal pain with palpation; therefore, this is not the most likely diagnosis in this case.
3. Internal hemorrhoids (most likely diagnosis)
   This is the most likely diagnosis, given the short duration of symptoms, the history of straining with a bowel movement, and the overall good health of the patient. On physical examination, you would expect the stool to be guaiac-negative, unless active bleeding is present.

MULTIPLE CHOICE

1. (A) Patient lying down on his or her side on the examining table
2. (B) Size
3. (D) Prostate cancer
4. (A) External hemorrhoids
5. (C) Rectal prolapse
6. (C) Herpes

Chapter 11: The Peripheral Vascular System

CASE STUDY

CASE STUDY: LEG PAIN

WHAT PARTS OF THE EXAM WOULD YOU LIKE TO PERFORM?

General Survey

Vital Signs

Skin

Cardiovascular

Abdomen

Peripheral Vascular/ Extremities

BASED ON THIS INFORMATION, WHAT IS YOUR DIFFERENTIAL DIAGNOSIS?

1. Deep venous thrombosis
   Deep venous thrombosis typically presents with edema of one lower extremity (as opposed to both). The edema is usually especially apparent in the calf. There may be erythema, warmth, and a tender palpable cord. Pulses are still palpable in the foot and ankle. Hair distribution is unaffected, since this is typically an acute presentation. When deep venous thrombosis is suspected, further testing is needed.

2. Lumbar spinal stenosis
   Lumbar spinal stenosis can result in calf, thigh, or buttock pain. The pain is typically not relieved by rest and may be worse with sitting upright, as this changes the angle of the spinal column and exerts more pressure on the peripheral nerves. The pain is relieved by leaning forward or by walking. Also, there are typically no skin changes or changes in peripheral pulses with spinal stenosis. Hyporeflexia may be present.

3. Peripheral vascular disease (most likely diagnosis)
   Mr. V.'s history suggests claudication, a symptom of peripheral vascular disease. In peripheral vascular disease, one or both lower extremities may be affected. Hair distribution is decreased. The skin is smooth and shiny. The toenails may be dystrophic. There is pallor on elevation of the extremity and rubor (redness) when the limb is dependent. There may be bruits over the abdominal aorta, iliac, femoral, carotid, or subclavian arteries. Pulses may be decreased or nonpalpable.

MULTIPLE CHOICE

1. (B) Lymphedema
2. (C) Allen's test
3. (B) Arterial insufficiency
4. (D) Venous insufficiency
5. (A) Orthostatic edema

MATCHING
ANATOMY

1. (D) Superficial veins: Great saphenous vein, small saphenous vein
2. (A) Deep veins: Femoral vein
3. (B) Location of arterial pulsations in the legs: Femoral artery, popliteal artery, dorsalis pedis artery, posterior tibial artery
4. (C) Location of arterial pulsations in the arms: Brachial artery, radial artery
5. (F) Drainage of epitrochlear lymph nodes: Ulnar surface of the forearm and hand, the little and ring fingers, and the adjacent surface of the middle finger
6. (E) Drainage of superficial inguinal lymph nodes: Superficial portions of the lower abdomen and buttock

TYPE AND DISTRIBUTION OF EDEMA

7. (C) Right-sided congestive heart failure: Dependent edema; sacral edema when patient is supine; may see increased JVP, enlarged liver, and enlarged heart; S3 present
8. (D) Hypoalbuminemia: Edema in the loose subcutaneous tissues of the eyelids; may also appear in the feet and legs

9. (B) Lymphedema: Localized edema; involves one or both legs
10. (A) Orthostatic edema: Edema of dependent areas; no cardiac or hepatic signs

Chapter 12: The Musculoskeletal System

CASE STUDIES

CASE STUDY: SHOULDER PAIN, ADULT

WHAT PARTS OF THE EXAM WOULD YOU LIKE TO PERFORM?

General Survey
Musculoskeletal – Neck and Shoulder

BASED ON THIS INFORMATION, WHAT IS YOUR DIFFERENTIAL DIAGNOSIS?

1. Cervical disc syndrome
   This disease is characterized by aching pain in the neck and shoulder with radicular pain in the arm; dermatomal loss of sensation or change in biceps jerk and triceps jerk may also be present. Our patient does not have aching pain in the neck, only the shoulder; also, she has no radicular symptoms to the arm. Therefore, this diagnosis is much less likely.
2. Bicipital tendonitis
   Bicipital tendonitis may resemble rotator cuff tendonitis and co-exist with it. Patients with bicipital tendonitis will also have weakness with abduction and forward flexion. However, our patient does not have tenderness to palpation in the bicipital groove.
3. Rotator cuff tear (most likely)
   Rotator cuff tears present with chronic, dull, aching pain with sharp pain during times of use. Repetitive use of the affected tendon is a precipitating factor. With her job as a floral designer, she will use motions that precipitate this pain. On physical examination, she has a positive drop arm test, which is very suggestive of a rotator cuff tear.

CASE STUDY: KNEE PAIN, ADULT

WHAT PARTS OF THE EXAM WOULD YOU LIKE TO PERFORM?

General Survey
Vital Signs
Skin
Musculoskeletal—Knee

BASED ON THIS INFORMATION, WHAT IS YOUR DIFFERENTIAL DIAGNOSIS?

1. Patellofemoral syndrome
   Characterized by a dull ache in the anterior knee with worsening pain during the first step that improves with continued walking. The pain is made worse by walking downward or after prolonged immobility. There are no specific physical examination findings, unlike the case of our patient, who has significant swelling in and around the knee and impaired range of motion.
2. Anterior cruciate ligament (ACL) tear
   An ACL tear is precipitated by a sudden trauma to the lower leg with the foot planted. In the case of our patient, this could have occurred; however, he states that he has had this same pain in the past and it has always improved with rest and icing of the knee. In the event of an ACL tear, the pain with the initial injury is much more dramatic and is unlikely to be something the patient would forget to tell the examiner. The pain of an ACL tear is worse with activity, and the patient may experience intermittent "giving way" of the knee. Our patient states that his knee feels unstable, but he has not experienced any episodes of it giving way. Additionally, he feels a clicking. His anterior drawer and Lachman's tests are negative, which makes the possibility of an ACL tear much less likely.
3. Meniscus tear (most likely diagnosis)
   The patient has experienced the same pain in the past, but it is more intense this time. The pain is sharp with occasional locking of the knee. The pain is worse with flexion of the affected knee, and patients may experience a clicking sensation. The McMurray's and Apley's tests are positive, which are diagnostic for meniscal tears.

CASE STUDY: NECK PAIN

WHAT PARTS OF THE EXAM WOULD YOU LIKE TO PERFORM?

> General Survey
>
> Vital Signs
>
> Skin
>
> Head and Neck
>
> Musculoskeletal
>
> Nervous System

BASED ON THIS INFORMATION, WHAT IS YOUR DIFFERENTIAL DIAGNOSIS?

1. Tension headache

   A tension headache is characterized by a pressing or tightening quality in the head of mild or moderate intensity and is bilateral. Patients often describe the feeling as "bandlike" around the temples. The pain occurs independently of a history of trauma and is not aggravated by routine physical activity. The neurologic examination is unremarkable. Tension headache is not the most likely diagnosis for Mrs. O. because she describes neck pain, not headache, and she has a history of whiplash.

2. Cervical spinal stenosis

   Cervical spinal stenosis arises from degenerative changes in the cervical vertebrae that encroach on the cervical spinal cord or nerve roots. Cervical spinal stenosis may occur without disc herniation. The pain develops slowly over time (years), is not continuous, and is related to an activity. There may be numbness and tingling of the upper arms bilaterally. Relief of symptoms with cervical traction is common. Typically, there is no history of repetitive motion or trauma as an initiating factor in the symptoms.

3. Cervical muscle spasm (most likely diagnosis)

   Ms. O. reports a history of overuse injury, which was then aggravated by a whiplash-type injury following a motor vehicle accident. Acute episodes are associated with pain, decreased mobility of the cervical spine, and paraspinal muscle spasm, resulting in stiffness of the neck and loss of motion. Muscle trigger points can often be localized. There are no focal neurologic findings. Neck pain or tenderness over the cervical vertebrae or paraspinal muscles after trauma warrants radiologic study.

CASE STUDY: LOW BACK PAIN

Note: It is useful to categorize causes of back pain as "on the midline" and "off the midline." "On the midline" causes include herniated disc, compression fracture, and metastasis. "Off the midline" causes include sacroiliitis, trochanteric bursitis, and hip arthritis.

WHAT PARTS OF THE EXAM WOULD YOU LIKE TO PERFORM?

> General Survey
>
> Vital Signs
>
> Skin
>
> Musculoskeletal
>
> Nervous System

BASED ON THIS INFORMATION, WHAT IS YOUR DIFFERENTIAL DIAGNOSIS?

1. Sacroiliitis

   Sacroiliitis is characterized by lumbosacral pain that radiates to the buttocks (most common), groin, or posterior thigh. The pain is aggravated by extensive use of the leg (such as walking). The pain may be reproduced by forced flexion of one lower extremity, coupled with extension and abduction of the other. There is tenderness with palpation of the sacroiliac joint. (Our patient does not have any tenderness over the S1 joint line, making sacroiliitis a less likely diagnosis in her case.) Sacroiliitis is frequently associated with other systemic illnesses such as ankylosing spondylitis, Reiter's syndrome (uveitis, arthritis, and urethritis), and inflammatory bowel disease.

2. Trochanteric bursitis

   Trochanteric bursitis is characterized by pain on palpation over the greater trochanter. The pain is located in the lateral hip and is often aggravated by weight bearing, rising from a chair, and climbing or descending stairs. The patient may note increased pain when lying on the affected side at night; some patients may be unable to walk due to severe pain. On physical examination, there is focal tenderness over the greater trochanter of the femur, and the pain may be elicited or aggravated by forced adduction. Internal and external rotation of the hip is preserved. Because our patient has no focal tenderness over the trochanteric bursa, trochanteric bursitis is not the most likely diagnosis.

3. Herniated disc (most likely diagnosis)

This condition is also known as herniated nucleus pulposus. A herniated disc is characterized by the sudden onset of back and leg pain. There are usually prior episodes of back pain. A flexion–rotation type of injury is typical. The pain is aggravated by flexion, sitting, or the Valsalva maneuver and is relieved by extension. By contrast, the pain of low back (lumbar) strain is aggravated by standing and twisting motions. Ms. Z.'s positive straight-leg raise test increases suspicion for a herniated disk. (To perform this test, the examiner passively extends the patient's knee and asks about discomfort. A straight-leg raise test is considered positive when pain radiates into the leg with extension of less than 60 degrees.) More than 95% of herniated discs are located at L4-L5 or L5-S1. Sometimes, the only symptom may be leg pain if there is a far lateral disc herniation. The neurologic examination may reveal focal abnormalities of strength, sensation, or reflexes.

MULTIPLE CHOICE

1. (D) Temporomandibular joint dysfunction
2. (A) Drop arm test
3. (C) Lateral epicondylitis
4. (A) Tinel's test
5. (B) Rheumatoid arthritis
6. (D) Osteoarthritis
7. (C) Scoliosis
8. (A) Compression fracture
9. (B) Anterior cruciate ligament tear
10. (C) Plantar fasciitis

MATCHING

1. (F) Synovial joint: Freely movable
2. (C) Cartilaginous joint: Slightly movable
3. (E) Fibrous joint: Immovable
4. (B) Spheroidal joint: Wide-ranging motion
5. (D) Hinge joint: Motion in one plane
6. (A) Condylar joint: Movement of two articulating surfaces

Chapter 13: The Nervous System: Mental Status

CASE STUDY

CASE STUDY: INCREASING CONFUSION

WHAT PARTS OF THE EXAM WOULD YOU LIKE TO PERFORM?

General Survey

Vital Signs

Skin

Head and Neck

Thorax and Lungs

Cardiovascular

Abdomen

Anus, Rectum, and Prostate

Peripheral Vascular/ Extremities

Musculoskeletal

Nervous System

BASED ON THIS INFORMATION, WHAT IS YOUR DIFFERENTIAL DIAGNOSIS?

1. Depression with acute psychosis

   Typically, the history of depression in some elderly patients is that of declining function (inability to carry out activities of daily living) over weeks, with changes in behavior. Patients may exhibit more anger and aggression, as opposed to sadness and tearfulness. Findings suggesting infection (e.g., hypotension, tachycardia) would not be expected.

2. New cerebrovascular accident (stroke)

   Although a cerebrovascular accident could be responsible for Mr. X.'s change in demeanor, he shows no evidence of motor deficits or other focal neurologic findings. To make this diagnosis, continued observation over the next 48 hours would be necessary to assess mental status and any changes in neurologic findings. Additionally, the patient's hydration status must be corrected, and other potential causes of his change in behavior (e.g., infection) must be excluded.

3. Dehydration and urosepsis (most likely diagnosis)

   In patients with dehydration, there may be altered mental status, lethargy, lightheadedness, or syncope. In general, mild dehydration produces reduced skin turgor, dry mucous membranes, and orthostatic hypotension. Moderate dehydration produces these symptoms, as well as oliguria or anuria, confusion, and resting hypotension. Severe hypotension produces shock or near shock. The patient has a history consistent with this diagnosis, but he also has a low temperature, which is more indicative of an infection. In the elderly patient, frequently more than one condition co-exists, and a search for infectious causes should also be pursued. Many elderly patients with urosepsis may not have dysuria, urinary frequency, or flank pain. There may be new onset of urinary incontinence or urinary retention. There may be fever or hypothermia. Confusion and delirium are also presenting signs.

MULTIPLE CHOICE

1. (B) Lethargic
2. (D) Delusion
3. (A) Calculating ability
4. (A) Dysarthria
5. (C) Orientation is fairly well maintained but becomes impaired in later stages of illness
6. (B) Obtunded

Chapter 14: The Nervous System: Cranial Nerves, Motor, Sensory, and Reflexes

CASE STUDIES

CASE STUDY: LOSS OF VISION

WHAT PARTS OF THE EXAM WOULD YOU LIKE TO PERFORM?

> General Survey
> Vital Signs
> Skin
> Eyes
> Musculoskeletal
> Neurologic

BASED ON THIS INFORMATION, WHAT IS YOUR DIFFERENTIAL DIAGNOSIS?

1. Conversion disorder

   The patient is a highly educated woman who appears to be coping well with her multiple stressors. She has never been diagnosed with depression nor had problems with her daily functioning—she has completed a master's degree, works full-time, and is a parent. Conversion disorder is more likely to be seen in patients with a lower level of education and those who have limited insight into their problems.

2. Stroke – Ischemic optic neuropathy

   Our patient is only 32 years old. She has no chronic medical conditions that would make the examiner concerned about ischemic disease in general.

3. Multiple sclerosis – Optic neuritis (most likely)
   Optic neuritis consists of a classic triad of unilateral loss of vision, eye pain, and dyschromatopsia (distorted color vision), with which our patient presents. Visual problems are the presenting sign in 50% of patients who are eventually diagnosed with multiple sclerosis, the most common problem of which is optic neuritis (25%); therefore, she would need to go through a more extensive work-up in both the physical examination as well as in diagnostic testing to look for this disease.

CASE STUDY: DIZZINESS

WHAT PARTS OF THE EXAM WOULD YOU LIKE TO PERFORM?

General Survey

Vital Signs

Skin

Head and Neck

Thorax and Lungs

Cardiovascular

Peripheral Vascular/ Extremities

Musculoskeletal

Nervous System

BASED ON THIS INFORMATION, WHAT IS YOUR DIFFERENTIAL DIAGNOSIS?

1. Meniere's disease
   This is a condition characterized by paroxysms of tinnitus, vertigo, pressure in the ear, and temporary hearing loss. Patients may describe the pressure in the ear as "feeling like the ear is full of water." The sensation of pressure in the ear may occur 1 to 2 days before the onset of the vertigo. The tinnitus may be described as a roar, hiss, or buzzing in the ear. The episodes can last minutes to hours; they decrease in frequency after multiple attacks and may return months to years later. Our patient does not have tinnitus, nor does she have a sensation of fullness in her ear. Therefore, it is less likely that she has Meniere's disease.

2. Acoustic neuroma
   An acoustic neuroma is a benign tumor of the eighth cranial nerve. In our patient's case, this diagnosis is less likely, given the relation of her symptoms to a preceding upper respiratory infection. The most common symptoms of an acoustic neuroma are progressive or sudden unilateral sensorineural hearing loss, tinnitus, and vertigo. Other symptoms include loss of balance, loss of facial sensation, or loss of function of the facial muscles or the muscles of mastication.

3. Vestibular neuronitis (most likely diagnosis)
   Our patient's presentation is typical of that of a patient with vestibular neuronitis. Patients usually complain of an abrupt onset of severe, debilitating vertigo with associated unsteadiness, nausea, and vomiting. They often describe their vertigo as a sensation that either they or their surroundings are spinning. Vertigo increases with head movement. Upon physical examination, spontaneous, unidirectional, horizontal nystagmus is the most important physical finding. The nystagmus is characterized by fast-phase oscillations beating toward the healthy ear. The nystagmus may be positional and apparent only when gazing toward the healthy ear, or it may be elicited by asking the patient to perform a Dix-Hallpike maneuver. (In this test, the patient sits in an upright position with his or her head turned 30 degrees to the side. The patient is rapidly moved from the sitting to the supine position with his or her head hanging in a dependent position over the edge of the examining table.) Viral infection of the vestibular nerve, the labyrinth, or both is believed to be the most common cause of vestibular neuronitis.

MULTIPLE CHOICE

1. (B) Brudzinski's sign
2. (A) Kernig's sign
3. (A) Pupils equal and reactive to light, pinpoint
4. (D) Brain abscess
5. (B) Bell's palsy
6. (C) S1
7. (D) CN XII (hypoglossal)

MATCHING

TERMINOLOGY

1. (E) Level of consciousness: Alertness and state of awareness of the environment
2. (D) Attention: Ability to focus or concentrate over time on one task or activity
3. (B) Recent memory: Ability to retain information over an interval of minutes, hours, or days
4. (C) Remote memory: Ability to retain information over an interval of years
5. (A) Orientation: Awareness of who or what the person is in relation to time, place, and people

CRANIAL NERVES

6. (F) CN I (olfactory): Smell
7. (D) CN II (optic): Vision
8. (K) CN III (oculomotor): Visual acuity, visual fields, ocular fundi, pupillary reactions
9. (E) CN IV (trochlear): Downward, inward movement of the eye
10. (G) CN V (trigeminal): Jaw movement; sensation of the face
11. (I) CN VI (abducens): Lateral deviation of the eye
12. (H) CN VII (facial): Facial movements, including facial expression, eye closure, and mouth closure
13. (J) CN VIII (vestibulocochlear): Hearing and balance
14. (B) CN IX (glossopharyngeal): Pharyngeal movement; sensation on the eardrum, ear canal, pharynx, and posterior tongue
15. (C) CN X (vagus): Movement of the palate, pharynx, and larynx
16. (L) CN XI (accessory): Shoulder and neck movements
17. (A) CN XII (hypoglossal): Tongue symmetry and position

REFLEXES

18. (H) Ankle reflex: S1
19. (A) Knee reflex: L2, L3, L4
20. (D) Brachioradialis: C3, C4
21. (F) Biceps: C5, C6
22. (G) Triceps: C6, C7
23. (E) Lower abdominal reflex: T10, T11, T12
24. (C) Upper abdominal reflex: T8, T9, T10
25. (B) Plantar reflex: L5, S1

MUSCLE ACTIONS

26. (F) Elbow flexion (biceps): C5, C6
27. (D) Elbow extension (triceps): C6, C7, C8
28. (B) Wrist extension: C6, C7, C8, radial nerve
29. (E) Grip strength: C7, C8, T1
30. (C) Finger abduction: C8, T1, ulnar nerve
31. (G) Thumb opposition: C8, T1, median nerve
32. (A) Hip flexion (iliopsoas): L2, L3, L4
33. (A) Hip adduction (adductors): L2, L3, L4
34. (H) Hip abduction (gluteus medius and minimus): L4, L5, S1
35. (J) Hip extension (gluteus maximus): S1
36. (A) Knee extension (quadriceps): L2, L3, L4
37. (I) Knee flexion (hamstrings): L4, L5, S1, S2
38. (K) Ankle dorsiflexion: L4, L5
39. (J) Ankle plantar flexion: S1

Chapter 15: Infants through Adolescents

CASE STUDY

CASE STUDY: WHEEZING, CHILD

WHAT PARTS OF THE EXAM WOULD YOU LIKE TO PERFORM?

General Survey

Vital Signs

Skin

Head and Neck

Thorax and Lungs

Cardiovascular (limited)

BASED ON THIS INFORMATION, WHAT IS YOUR DIFFERENTIAL DIAGNOSIS?

1. Foreign body

   There is no history of the patient ingesting a foreign body, although this could have occurred without the daycare worker or parent realizing it. The patient appears to be comfortable; children who ingest a foreign body would be in more pain. Also, there is no audible wheezing (i.e., audible without a stethoscope) or stridor. Children who ingest a foreign body in the respiratory tract typically exhibit wheezing, stridor, and difficulty breathing.

2. Respiratory syncytial virus (RSV) bronchiolitis

   Most affected children with RSV bronchiolitis have a history of exposure to older children or adults with minor respiratory diseases within the week preceding the onset of illness, and they usually experience a mild upper respiratory tract infection with clear nasal discharging and sneezing for several days prior to the onset of wheezing. The fever range is 101–102°F, and mild symptoms resolve spontaneously in 1–3 days. The peak age for RSV bronchiolitis is 2–6 months, although it can occur from the newborn time period up until age 2. Our patient is older than this typical age range, and he does not have a fever, so the diagnosis of RSV bronchiolitis is much less likely

3. Asthma (most likely diagnosis)

   The patient has a paroxysmal cough, worse at night, which is one of the presenting signs of asthma in this age group. He also has symptoms of either a respiratory infection or allergies, and he has a dog in his household, all of which are considered to be precipitants of an asthma attack. His family history of asthma and allergic rhinitis also goes along with the diagnosis of asthma.

Chapter 16: The Pregnant Woman

MULTIPLE CHOICE

1. (A) You reassure her that pregnancy-related nausea usually only lasts for the first trimester and that most likely her nausea and appetite will improve soon
2. (D) You reassure her that this is a normal part of pregnancy because the hormones are causing relaxation of the joints and ligaments, which changes the normal curvature of the lower spine
3. (B) Cyanotic cervical os; soft to palpation
4. (A) The patient will feel the baby move
5. (B) Leopold's maneuvers

MATCHING

1. (B) EDC: Date of delivery
2. (D) LMP: Most recent onset of menses
3. (A) Nägele's rule: Calculation to determine expected date of confinement
4. (C) Leopold's maneuvers: Technique to determine size and position of the fetus

Chapter 17: The Older Adult

CASE STUDIES

CASE STUDY: URINARY INCONTINENCE

WHAT PARTS OF THE EXAM WOULD YOU LIKE TO PERFORM?

General Survey

Vital Signs

Abdomen (limited)
Genitourinary
Musculoskeletal
Neurologic

BASED ON THIS INFORMATION, WHAT IS YOUR DIFFERENTIAL DIAGNOSIS?

1. Urinary tract infection
   Losing control of bladder function may be one symptom of infection in this age group; however, she denies burning pain with urination, hematuria, incomplete emptying, and urinary hesitancy, which are symptoms frequently associated with infection. Her problem is worse with coughing and sneezing, which is not typical of an infectious process. Her symptoms are chronic, which is also atypical for an infectious process. Urinary tract infection can make other forms of incontinence worse.

2. Functional incontinence
   Functional incontinence by definition involves no anatomic or pathologic disease process. People with functional incontinence may have problems thinking, moving, or communicating that prevent them from reaching a toilet. Functional incontinence may be temporary, as in hip surgery patients in the postoperative phase when they are not allowed to be weight bearing and have to rely on someone else to help them get to the restroom. Functional incontinence can occur routinely in patients with dementia, since it is difficult for them to communicate the need to go to the bathroom. Our patient is able to give a coherent history and is still physically active; therefore, she is much less likely to have the diagnosis of functional incontinence.

3. Stress urinary incontinence (most likely diagnosis)
   Stress incontinence is defined as inability to control urination when pressure is exerted on the bladder. This type of incontinence is precipitated by any activity that increases abdominal pressure: laughing, sneezing, coughing, lifting, jogging, etc. Women have increased susceptibility if they have had a hysterectomy, gone through menopause, or had multiple vaginal deliveries. Our patient has all of the risk factors: female, menopause, posthysterectomy, and history of multiple vaginal births. She also has atrophic vaginitis, which is a comorbid condition associated with stress incontinence.

CASE STUDY: MEMORY LOSS

WHAT PARTS OF THE EXAM WOULD YOU LIKE TO PERFORM?

General Survey
Vital Signs
Head and Neck (limited)
Cardiovascular (limited)
Neurologic
Mental Status

BASED ON THIS INFORMATION, WHAT IS YOUR DIFFERENTIAL DIAGNOSIS?

1. Hypothyroidism
   The presentation of hypothyroidism is atypical in elderly patients. They may complain of fatigue or sluggishness. They may experience weight gain, dry skin, or constipation. On physical examination, in advanced hypothyroidism, they may appear to have a flat affect and have doughy skin from myxedema. They may have a heart murmur or swelling in their lower extremities, or delayed Achilles reflex return phase. Our patient denies fatigue, weight changes, dry skin, and constipation. On examination, she does appear to have a flat affect, but she has no significant physical findings that are consistent with hypothyroidism. To truly exclude this problem, further testing is needed.

2. Depressive disorder
   She has recently lost her spouse of >60 years; she does admit to being sad and lonely. These findings are compatible with depression. The SIG E CAPS mnemonic can be used to help the clinician remember all of the symptoms of depression to ask about:

- Sleep increase or decrease
- Interest diminished in formerly pleasurable activities
- Guilt or low self-esteem

- Energy loss
- Concentration impaired
- Appetite changes
- Psychomotor agitation or retardation
- Suicidal ideation

> In the elderly, less typical presentations include headaches, stomach aches, or chronic pain; also, they may have memory problems. The somatic complaints and memory loss makes the diagnosis of depression more difficult. Our patient denies headaches, stomach aches, and chronic pain; she does not admit to having memory problems—her daughter is the one who brought her in. With depression, the patient is aware of his or her memory difficulty, whereas our patient has no insight into this problem. Therefore, this is less likely to be the diagnosis, but could be a complicating factor.

3. Dementia (most likely diagnosis)
   Signs and symptoms of dementia include gradually increasing memory loss, confusion, unclear thinking including losing problem-solving skills, agitated behavior or delusions, becoming lost in formerly familiar circumstances, and loss of interest in daily or usual activities. Spouses often cover for the memory deficits of their spouse, and the children only realize that there is a problem when that spouse dies, which has occurred in this patient's case. Now that Catherine's husband has died, there is no one to keep her in a routine, prepare her meals, or take her to her usual activities. The mental status examination is one of the most important parts of the examination in this case. The questions that were asked in this case are included in the Folstein Mini-Mental State Exam, and, if the entire form were completed, there would be a significant low score. This is one indication that the patient has dementia and not depression. This is the most likely diagnosis for this case.

CASE STUDY: ABNORMAL GAIT

WHAT PARTS OF THE EXAM WOULD YOU LIKE TO PERFORM?

General Survey

Vital Signs

Head and Neck (limited—looking for central causes of gait abnormality)

Cardiovascular (limited—looking for murmurs or arrhythmias)

Peripheral Vascular

Musculoskeletal

Neurologic

BASED ON THIS INFORMATION, WHAT IS YOUR DIFFERENTIAL DIAGNOSIS?

1. Lumbar disc disease
   Lumbar disc disorders are characterized by sharp or numbing pain located in the midline or paraspinal area of the lower back with radiation of pain into the buttocks or posterior thigh. Our patient does not have these symptoms. Her problem is progressive over several months, as opposed to lumbar disc disease, which, unless there is neurologic compromise (bowel or bladder incontinence, reduced strength or reflexes on physical examination), is self-limited with months to years between exacerbations.
2. Osteoarthritis
   The pain of osteoarthritis is that of dull aching over affected joint areas, usually located in the knees, hips, base of thumb, spine, and shoulders. The pain is worse after use of the joint, and there may be morning stiffness that lasts less than 30 minutes and that improves with activity. The pain and problems with balance (if arthritis is in the knees or hips) is worse with repetitive motion or strain on the joint. The clinical course is progressive with intermittent flares. Our patient does not have pain in her muscles or joints, nor does she have morning stiffness.
3. Parkinson's disease (most likely diagnosis)
   Parkinson's disease is characterized by a resting tremor, bradykinesia, and rigidity of the extremities. Initial presenting signs may simply be constitutional: increased fatigue or general malaise along with increased irritability or depression. The family may notice changes sooner than the patient, such as lack of facial expression and animation or slower, stiffer, unsteadier movements. The "get up and go" test is described in the neurologic examination section and reveals retropulsion (backward movement when initiating gait) as well as

bradykinesia. Our patient also has a resting tremor that goes away when she is asked to perform the finger-to-nose and Romberg maneuvers. She does not yet have rigidity of the extremities. The diagnosis of Parkinson's disease is made over time, using your history taking and physical examination. Diagnostic tests are used to exclude other diseases.

MULTIPLE CHOICE

1. (B) Diastolic blood pressure increases with aging, although it stops rising at about the sixth decade
2. (B) As people age, the pacemaker cells decline in the sinoatrial node; the older adult is more likely to have abnormal heart rhythms, and a pause for every third beat is one type of ectopy; an electrocardiogram is needed to confirm this pattern
3. (B) The lens loses its elasticity over time, and the eye is less able to accommodate and focus on near objects; therefore, the patient will be expected to have blurring of near vision
4. (B) Human speech is considered to be a middle-ranged sound, and, during the aging process, there is a loss of acuity, starting with high-pitched sounds but extending to the middle range and then into the low range.
5. (C) The aortic valve cusps thicken with fibrous tissue as part of the aging process, which in turn results in calcifications. The aortic valve leaflets then become immobile, which results in the heart sounds heard in aortic stenosis
6. (A) The patient most likely has atrophic vaginitis, which results in an increased pallor of the vaginal mucosa, which would normally be pink.
7. (A) The patient has a normal mini-mental state examination score; she does not have symptoms or signs of depression or of infection; therefore, this is the most correct answer.
8. (C) This is a common presentation of acute myocardial infarction in the elderly.
9. (C) Falls are an example of a geriatric syndrome, which is characterized by the interaction and probable synergism among multiple risk factors.
10. (D) This is an activity of daily living; it represents basic self-care ability.